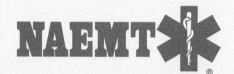

THIRD ED

M000248797

Geriatric Education
for Emergency Medical Services

COURSE MANUAL

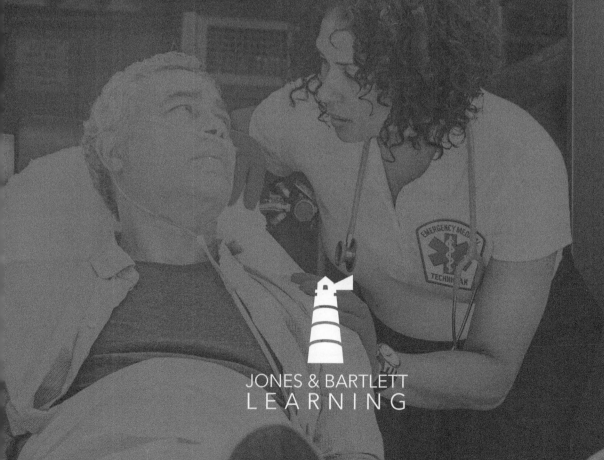

JONES & BARTLETT
LEARNING

World Headquarters
Jones & Bartlett Learning
25 Mall Road
Burlington, MA 01803
978-443-5000
info@jblearning.com
www.jblearning.com
www.psglearning.com

Jones & Bartlett Learning books and products are available through most bookstores and online booksellers. To contact the Jones & Bartlett Learning Public Safety Group directly, call 800-832-0034, fax 978-443-8000, or visit our website, www.psglearning.com.

Substantial discounts on bulk quantities of Jones & Bartlett Learning publications are available to corporations, professional associations, and other qualified organizations. For details and specific discount information, contact the special sales department at Jones & Bartlett Learning via the above contact information or send an email to specialsales@jblearning.com.

Copyright © 2024 by the National Association of Emergency Medical Technicians

All rights reserved. No part of the material protected by this copyright may be reproduced or utilized in any form, electronic or mechanical, including photocopying, recording, or by any information storage and retrieval system, without written permission from the copyright owner.

The content, statements, views, and opinions herein are the sole expression of the respective authors and not that of Jones & Bartlett Learning, LLC. Reference herein to any specific commercial product, process, or service by trade name, trademark, manufacturer, or otherwise does not constitute or imply its endorsement or recommendation by Jones & Bartlett Learning, LLC and such reference shall not be used for advertising or product endorsement purposes. All trademarks displayed are the trademarks of the parties noted herein. *Geriatric Education for Emergency Medical Services, Third Edition Course Manual* is an independent publication and has not been authorized, sponsored, or otherwise approved by the owners of the trademarks or service marks referenced in this product.

There may be images in this book that feature models; these models do not necessarily endorse, represent, or participate in the activities represented in the images. Any screenshots in this product are for educational and instructive purposes only. Any individuals and scenarios featured in the case studies throughout this product may be real or fictitious but are used for instructional purposes only.

The procedures and protocols in this book are based on the most current recommendations of responsible medical sources. The National Association of Emergency Medical Technicians (NAEMT) and the publisher, however, make no guarantee as to, and assume no responsibility for, the correctness, sufficiency, or completeness of such information or recommendations. Other or additional safety measures may be required under particular circumstances.

This textbook is intended solely as a guide to the appropriate procedures to be employed when rendering emergency care to the sick and injured. It is not intended as a statement of the standards of care required in any particular situation, because circumstances and the patient's physical condition can vary widely from one emergency to another. Nor is it intended that this textbook shall in any way advise emergency personnel concerning legal authority to perform the activities or procedures discussed. Such local determination should be made only with the aid of legal counsel.

29041-7

Production Credits
Vice President, Product Management: Marisa R. Urbano
Vice President, Content Strategy and Implementation: Christine Emerton
Director, Product Management: Laura Carney
Director, Content Management: Donna Gridley
Manager, Content Strategy: Tiffany Sliter
Content Strategist: Alex Belloli
Content Coordinator: Mark Restuccia
Director, Project Management and Content Services: Karen Scott
Manager, Project Management: Jackie Reynen
Project Manager: Erin Bosco
Program Manager: Rachel DiMaggio

Senior Digital Project Specialist: Angela Dooley
Director, Marketing: Brian Rooney
Content Services Manager: Colleen Lamy
Product Fulfillment Manager: Wendy Kilborn
Composition: S4Carlisle Publishing Services
Cover/Text Design: Scott Moden
Senior Media Development Editor: Troy Liston
Rights & Permissions Manager: John Rusk
Rights Specialist: Liz Kincaid
Cover Image (Title Page): © Tammy Hanratty/Corbis/VCG/ Corbis/Getty Images
Printing and Binding: Sheridan Kentucky

Library of Congress Cataloging-in-Publication Data

LCCN: 2023007822

6048

Printed in the United States of America

26 25 24 23   10 9 8 7 6 5 4 3 2 1

Brief Contents

Table of Contents

Chapter 14 Urinary Catheter and Colostomy Bag Care....................171

Chapter 15 Implantable Cardioverter Defibrillators.......................183

Preface

Due to longer life expectancies and advances in medical care, the geriatric population is the largest growing population group on the planet. Globally, the number of people 80 years of age and older is expected to triple by 2050 (from 143 million to 426 million). Yet even with improvements in medical care, geriatric patients account for approximately 40% of all emergency medical services (EMS) calls in the United States. For EMS practitioners responding to those calls, NAEMT is proud to offer the third edition of *Geriatric Education for Emergency Medical Services (GEMS) Course Manual*.

The GEMS program was developed to provide practitioners with an understanding of the need for a comprehensive assessment of geriatric patients. Because the aging process affects all body systems, the course provides an overview of changes that occur as we age and how those changes can impact patient presentation. Completing a full assessment that integrates and responds to differences in geriatric pathophysiology is critical to recognizing and responding quickly and effectively to the critically ill and/or injured older adult. Incorporating the GEMS Diamond (Geriatric, Environmental, Medical, and Social assessments) can help practitioners formulate a holistic diagnostic and treatment approach for older patients.

This third edition of GEMS incorporates a new case-based approach to recognition of common medical disorders, updated content to reflect evidence-based guidelines in current practice, optional lessons on patient medical devices, and this new GEMS course manual. The course manual is designed to be a resource for students that can be consulted after the course to help them provide the best care for older adults in each community.

The NAEMT GEMS author team

Acknowledgments

GEMS Course Medical Director

Sue A. Schemel, MD, FACEP
Adjunct Clinical Assistant Professor of Emergency Medicine
Touro College of Osteopathic Medicine
Middletown, New York

GEMS Course Author Team

Kelly Kohler, MS, Paramedic, CCP-C, CHSE, NCEE
Member, AMLS Committee
Assistant Professor of EMS, Touro College of Osteopathic
    Medicine
Assistant Professor of EMS, Dutchess Community College
Paramedic, Empress EMS
Poughkeepsie, New York

Jeff J. Messerole, EMT-P
Immediate Past Chair, AMLS Committee
PHTLS and AMLS Affiliate Faculty
Spirit Lake, Iowa

Jarrod Nall, AAS, Paramedic, CCP-C
AMLS and GEMS Affiliate Faculty
Clinical Manager, LifeNet, Inc.
Texarkana, Texas

Joanne Piccininni, MBA, NRP, MICP
Chair, PHT Committee
Program Director, Assistant Professor
Bergen Community College Paramedic Science Program
Lyndhurst, New Jersey

John Shanley, NQEMT-EMT
PHTLS Faculty
Training Coordinator, Medical Ambulance Service/Medical
    Emergency Medical Training
Dublin, Ireland

NAEMT Editorial Director

Nancy Hoffmann, MSW
Senior Director, Education Publishing
National Association of Emergency
Medical Technicians

GEMS Course Manual Writer

Jim McKendry, BSc, MEM, ACP (Retired)
Winnipeg, Manitoba, Canada

GEMS Course Manual Editor

Kristen Lovell
Education Editor
National Association of Emergency
Medical Technicians
St. Louis, Missouri

GEMS Course Contributors

Terri King, NRP, AAS, BS, MA
EPC Affiliate Faculty
Division Commander Clinical Practice
Williamson County EMS
Georgetown, Texas

CHAPTER 1

Changes with Age and Assessment of the Older Patient

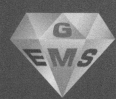

LESSON OBJECTIVES

- Discuss anatomical and physiologic changes of the aging population.
- Recognize challenges to and strategies for effective communication with geriatric patients.
- List barriers to care that may affect the geriatric patient.
- Identify the components of the GEMS Diamond.
- Demonstrate integration of the GEMS Diamond within the primary survey and management of geriatric patients.
- Explain the purpose of ongoing assessment.

Introduction

The **geriatric** age group is generally considered age 65 years and older; however, most older persons do not require geriatric medical care until between ages 70 and 80. The typical EMS practitioner is younger than 65 years of age. Therefore, comprehending, appreciating, and empathizing with the aging and medical complexities facing an older patient may be challenging for EMS practitioners.

EMS practitioner exposure to geriatric patients is increasing. Advances in science and technology have increased average human life expectancy across the globe. Consequently, the proportion of the world's population older than 65 years is rising. The United Nations notes that the fastest growing age group in the world is older adults. Already (since 2018), adults older than 65 years outnumber children younger than 5 years, and by 2050, they are expected to outnumber adolescents as well. In 2015, the geriatric population comprised approximately 8.5% of the world's population. This number is estimated to increase to 12% by 2030 and 16.7% by 2050. In the United States, the geriatric portion of the population grew from 12.4% in 2000 to 16.0% in 2018.

According to the Centers for Disease Control and Prevention, improved health care in the United States is largely responsible for increasing life expectancy for a 65-year-old American from 11.9 more years in 2010 to 19.6 more years in 2019 (**FIGURE 1-1**).

An Older Crowd

The number of those aged 65 years and older in the United States is projected to surpass the number of those younger than 18 years by 2035 and grow to almost 90 million by 2050.

A Korean study published in 2020 observed the geriatric age group was more likely to use EMS when compared to younger adults. An American study conducted from 2010 to 2011 observed similar findings. In both studies, greater use of EMS as the patient's age increased was noted.

Comorbidity Complications

Ninety percent of those over 65 years are estimated to have one or more chronic medical conditions such as diabetes, heart disease, arthritis, and anxiety or depression.

Understanding the physical, physiologic, and psychological challenges faced by older patients is required to provide empathetic and appropriate care. And yet, when surveyed, EMS practitioners perceive a deficit in both initial and continuing prehospital education for care of older adults. Studies have shown that older patients are often undertriaged (transported to lower-level trauma centers or acute care facilities) by EMS practitioners when compared to younger patients, which significantly impacts mortality rates. Undertriaging may be influenced by the following factors:

- A higher number of comorbidities (risk of dangerous complications from comorbidities is raised, as patient may be triaged for the only chief complaint)
- Polypharmacy and drug interactions (antiplatelet or anticoagulant therapy impacting internal bleeding)
- Altered physiologic response (lack of fever in cases of infection, normal vital signs in the setting of hypoperfusion)
- Decreased ability to clearly explain symptoms (less information to use when determining differential diagnosis, possible altered mental status)
- An impaired capacity to heal (overall changes due to impact of aging on wound healing)
- Perceived significance of injury pattern (low-level falls can be more traumatic for older adults and require higher level of trauma center care)

Making EMS care more difficult is the differentiation in medical conditions experienced by older patients within a similar age range. To illustrate how this applies to emergency care, 20-year-olds often share a similar health status and social situations. In contrast, 80-year-olds usually have differing health conditions and levels of social interaction, ranging from independent living to requiring fully supportive care to perform activities of daily living.

Most Common Reasons for EMS Contact, Interventions Performed, and Medications Administered

Geriatric patients most commonly access EMS due to syncope, cardiac arrest, arrhythmias, cerebrovascular accident (stroke), and shock (due to conditions such as sepsis or dehydration). The most common EMS interventions for geriatric patients are establishing intravenous (IV) access, conducting 12-lead ECG assessment, performing CPR, and intubation. Commonly administered medications by EMS to this age group include epinephrine, atropine, furosemide, amiodarone, and albuterol or ipratropium.

Supporting Overall Well-Being

The World Health Organization (WHO) defines healthy aging as, "the process of developing and maintaining the functional ability that enables well-being in older age." Healthy aging does not mean that older adults are free of disease or limitations. Instead, it refers to creating various environments that enable functional abilities in older adults. Older adults may be experiencing bodily deterioration or chronic illness, but when those health conditions are under control, overall well-being is not impacted much.

Functional ability means a person is capable of being who they want to be and participating in activities that they value (**FIGURE 1-2**). It can include being mobile, meeting daily basic needs, learning and contributing to society, building and maintaining social relationships, growth as a person, and the capacity to make independent decisions. Functional ability is made

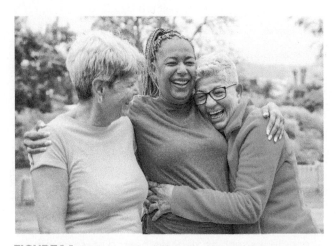

FIGURE 1-1 With improved life expectancies, there are more older adults than ever, and that population is growing.
© Sabrina Bracher/Shutterstock

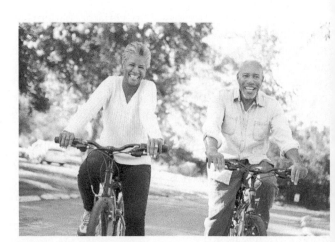

FIGURE 1-2 Older adults' functional ability depends on a supportive physical and emotional environment.
© Monkey Business Images/Shutterstock

up of the relevant aspects of a person's life, their own intrinsic capacity to function in meaningful ways, and how these two characteristics interact with each other.

Intrinsic capacity is the physical and mental capacities a person has available to use in daily life, including the ability to think clearly, sensory input (seeing, hearing, tasting, feeling, smelling), memory recall, and mobility. In the aging population, intrinsic capacity is often affected to a greater degree than in the younger population due to the aging process itself, the presence of chronic disease, injury, physical ability, mental health factors, and more.

Critical Thinking Question

How does an older adult's environment affect their health?

Anatomy and Physiology of Aging

Everyone experiences the effects of aging differently due to variations in genetics, lifestyles, and diets. However, a common aspect of aging is that no body system will be spared decline. There are many theories on how the aging process occurs, as it is not well understood. The aging process has been defined in literature as the result of the buildup of toxic changes in cells and tissues over time that increases the risk of disease and cellular death. Understanding the changes due to aging is necessary for proper assessment and management of geriatric patients (**FIGURE 1-3**).

Remember that aging is not a disease that can be cured or prevented. Some geriatric patients in their 80s exhibit similar mental and physical capacities as persons in their 30s, yet some geriatric patients in their 80s may need more supportive care to perform basic **activities of daily living (ADLs)**. Basic activities of daily living include feeding oneself, walking, continence, toileting, dressing, and personal hygiene.

Why We Don't Live to 130 Years (Yet)

In general, body systems' operating efficiencies decline about 1% per year after age 30.

Respiratory System

Changes to the respiratory system are often variable due to differences in health status, life experiences, and lifestyle. Factors include chronic exposure to

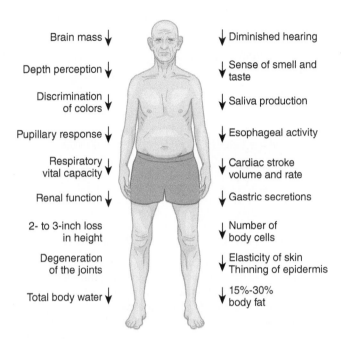

Brain mass ↓
Depth perception ↓
Discrimination of colors ↓
Pupillary response ↓
Respiratory vital capacity ↓
Renal function ↓
2- to 3-inch loss in height
Degeneration of the joints
Total body water ↓

↓ Diminished hearing
↓ Sense of smell and taste
↓ Saliva production
↓ Esophageal activity
↓ Cardiac stroke volume and rate
↓ Gastric secretions
↓ Number of body cells
↓ Elasticity of skin Thinning of epidermis
↓ 15%-30% body fat

FIGURE 1-3 Changes caused by aging.
Copyright © 2024 National Association of Emergency Medical Technicians (NAEMT).

environmental pollutants, repeated pulmonary infections, smoking, and socioeconomic factors. Tolerance of stressors from exertion or minor disease can be greatly reduced in the geriatric age group. For instance, a minor respiratory infection in an older patient can become life-threatening.

Lungs Age Quickly

Maximum levels of pulmonary function are reached by age 20 to 25 years and then progressively decline.

The airway of an older patient can be challenging to maintain. Weakened musculature of the upper airway can cause the tongue to fall back and other soft tissues of the upper airway to close more easily when the patient is fatigued or has an altered level of consciousness. Displaced dentures can lead to upper airway obstruction directly; or, along with loss of teeth, cause obstruction by aspiration of improperly chewed food. Decreased gag reflex also increases the risk of upper airway obstruction.

Loss of mechanisms that protect the lower airways also contributes to increased airway obstruction risk. Decreased cough reflex, loss of cilia, and increased mucous glands in the bronchioles play a part in this.

Muscles of the lower airway also weaken with age. This muscle loss causes the lower, smaller airways to

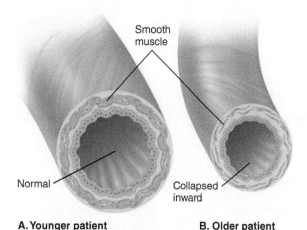

Smooth
muscle

Normal

Collapsed
inward

A. Younger patient

B. Older patient

FIGURE 1-4 A. Healthy muscle in the younger patient's airway helps maintain the open airway during the pressures of inhalation. **B.** Muscle weakening with age can lead to airway collapse that may produce wheezes.

© Jones & Bartlett Learning

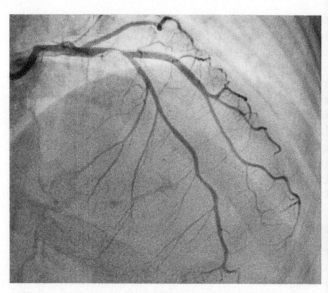

FIGURE 1-5 Angiography showing atherosclerosis/arterial stenosis.

© Pitchyfoto/Shutterstock

collapse more easily. Combined with a loss of elastic recoil in the alveoli, airway closure at high lung volumes results. This leads to less effective alveolar ventilation and increased **residual lung volume** (air remaining in the lungs following a normal exhalation). Skeletal muscles of the chest wall and diaphragm also weaken with age causing further reduction in ventilation. By the age of 75 years, the **vital lung capacity** (air volume maximally exhaled after maximal inhalation) is reduced by 50% (**FIGURE 1-4**).

Finally, sensitivity of the **chemoreceptors** in the aortic arch is reduced. These receptors trigger the brainstem to initiate ventilation. Decreased sensitivity and slowed impulse transmission from the brainstem to the diaphragm and intercostal muscles decrease arterial oxygen concentration. Pulse oximetry readings as low as 93% may be in the "normal" range for an older patient.

Cardiovascular System

Decline in cardiac health specifically associated with the aging process involves the deterioration of the cardiac tissue, cardiac conduction system, and vascular structure. The conduction system is responsible for determining the heart rate and coordinating the efficiency of cardiac tissue contraction. Irregularities in the conduction system (arrhythmias) become more common as physiologic changes due to aging affect its performance.

Due to normal cellular death, the pacemaker cells of the SA node are reduced by more than 90% by 70 years of age. Additionally, fibrosis and fatty deposits along the conduction pathway promote irregular

conduction resulting in arrhythmias. Changes in cellular function due to aging also cause a longer duration of cardiac contraction, which increases myocardial oxygen demand while simultaneously lowering the effectiveness of oxygen delivery to the myocardium.

Baroreceptors in the aortic arch and carotid sinus become less sensitive to changes in blood volume, causing widening pulse pressures, so blood pressure changes are slowed. Sitting upright from supine or standing from a supine or seated position can cause a decrease in systolic blood pressure known as **orthostatic hypotension**.

Vascular structural changes include left ventricular enlargement, aortic stenosis (narrowing), and aortic and mitral valve calcification. All these changes decrease the ability of the heart to efficiently pump blood. Vascular structural changes involve thickening and stiffening of the vessel walls, which results in hypertension and widening pulse pressures. These changes contribute to the development of **atherosclerosis**, which can lead to coronary heart disease. Atherosclerosis is a progressive disease primarily responsible for cardiac function decline during the aging process, and it affects more than 60% of people aged 65 years and older. (**FIGURE 1-5**)

Losing Heart

Fewer than 10% of SA node pacemaker cells remain by the age of 70 years. From the age of 17 to 90 years, 30% to 35% of myocardial cells are lost.

Nervous System

Aging changes to the nervous system are dramatic and often associated with age-related disability. Approximately 35% of those over the age of 70 years will have gait abnormalities and mobility problems.

Structurally, aging causes 5% to 50% of nerve cell loss and shrinkage of the remaining cells. This age-related loss and shrinkage of brain tissue results in a decrease of beneficial and restorative deep sleep. An estimated loss of 55% of short-term memory is also associated with brain tissue changes.

The physical decrease in brain size increases the space between the brain surface and the skull. Veins that cross this space become stretched and more easily torn when trauma to the head occurs. Because of this extra space, signs of increased intracranial pressure will be delayed when subdural bleeding is present.

Peripheral nerves also deteriorate over time. Peripheral sensations and reflexes slow, putting the older person at risk for injuries such as burns. Peripheral sensations may also be misinterpreted, which can make patient assessment more challenging.

Optic neuropathies may develop, potentially leading to overall decreased vision as well as a decreased field of vision.

Integumentary System

The most visible sign of aging involves changes to the integumentary system (**FIGURE 1-6**). Levels of elastin and collagen in the skin decrease with age, making the skin less elastic and weaker, respectively. Accessory organs of the integumentary system also succumb to the aging process. Hair follicles produce hair that is thinner and has less melanin resulting in gray, white, and silver hair color. Sebaceous glands produce less oil, so the skin also becomes drier. The result is wrinkled and more delicate skin. Thinning of the subcutaneous fat layer, as well as decreased sweat gland activity, inhibits the ability to regulate heat. These changes also mean the

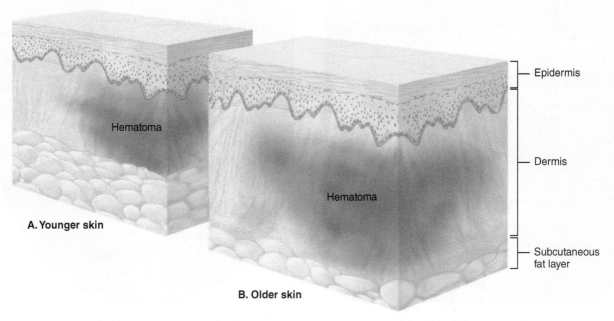

FIGURE 1-6 A. In younger skin, the tight interface between skin and the subcutaneous fat layer tends to control bleeding in subcutaneous injuries. **B.** The looser connection between skin and fat in older skin exerts less control on bleeding and may result in larger hematomas.

skin is injured more easily than in younger adults and is not able to control bleeding as well, which can lead to extensive hematomas and skin tears.

Critical Thinking Question

Why are older adults so prone to skin tears and pressure ulcers?

Musculoskeletal System

Degenerative changes to the musculoskeletal system of older adults vary by patient, but typically include progressive deterioration in physical ability and **osteoporosis**. Osteoporosis is the loss of bone mass when the rate of bone reabsorption is greater than the rate of new bone production. Bones become porous and brittle.

Osteoporosis leads to weakening of the skeletal structure and puts the older person at greater risk of bone fracture, spinal abnormalities including **kyphosis,** and limited range of motion (**FIGURE 1-7**). Two out of three patients will exhibit some degree of kyphosis (hunchback) due to atrophy of the supporting body structures.

These changes may lessen participation in physical activity, which causes further deterioration. Mobility is also negatively impacted by osteoporosis.

Osteoporosis and Fracture Risk

An estimated 40% of postmenopausal women and 30% of older men will suffer a fracture due to osteoporosis.

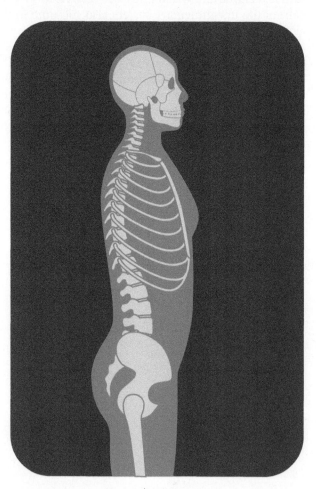
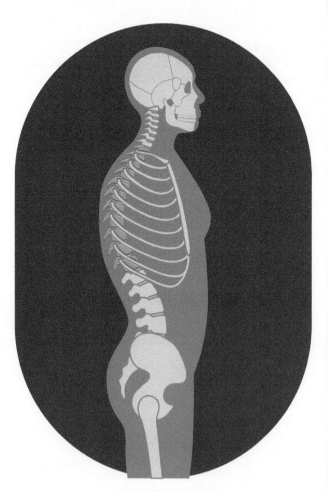

Normal spine   Kyphosis

FIGURE 1-7 A healthy spine is illustrated on the left. The image on the right shows kyphosis—a common spinal abnormality in older adults due to degenerative changes and osteoporosis.

Other tissues of the musculoskeletal system also deteriorate with age as muscle tissue shrinks and is lost and replaced by fat. Ligaments, tendons, and cartilage in the joints lose elasticity, and synovial fluid volume decreases. These changes lead to arthritis. The loss of muscle decreases strength, and increased fat alters how some medications affect geriatric patients.

Endocrine System

Diabetes mellitus is the most common endocrine disease in older persons, primarily type 2. This is due to increased insulin resistance and impaired pancreatic islet function that occur during the aging process. Older women more commonly have hyperparathyroidism, hypothyroidism, and hyperthyroidism. Fluid balance issues can occur with overproduction of antidiuretic hormone.

Though not an endocrine disorder itself, osteoporosis can be caused by common endocrine disorders. These disorders are the most frequent secondary cause of osteoporosis.

Diabetes: A Common Problem

By 2027, most of the American population with diabetes is anticipated to be over the age of 65 years. Approximately 26% of geriatric patients have a diagnosis of diabetes.

Gastrointestinal System

The smooth muscles of the gastrointestinal tract also weaken with age, resulting in decreased salivation, increased heartburn and gastric reflux (**FIGURE 1-8**), fecal incontinence, and constipation from diminished peristalsis and poor diet. Hepatic metabolism also slows down, causing drugs and other toxins to be metabolized at a slower rate, meaning the drugs can accumulate to potentially toxic levels.

GASTROESOPHAGEAL REFLUX DISEASE

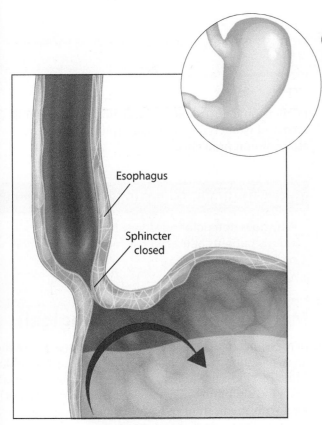

Esophagus

Sphincter closed

Healthy stomach

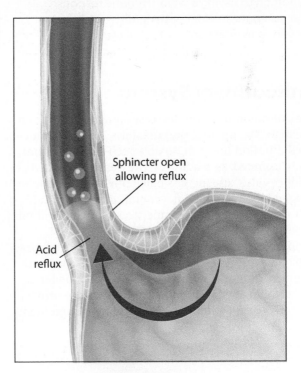

Sphincter open allowing reflux

Acid reflux

GERD stomach

FIGURE 1-8 Gastroesophageal reflux disease (GERD) is common in older adults due to deterioration of the muscle control of the esophageal sphincter.

Immune System

Normal cellular replacement that occurs with aging causes restructuring of the immune system. These changes allow infections to occur more easily while also weakening the protective response to pathogens. Generally, systemic and cellular immune responses become less effective and slower to respond. Older patients typically have chronic low-level inflammation due to poor immune response to continued exposure to antigens. Pneumonia and urinary tract infections are common in bed-bound and immobile patients, and they are at an increased risk of sepsis.

The aging population is also less responsive to vaccines, has more symptomatic illness when infected, and experiences longer recovery times. These changes increase the risk of severe disease when exposed to pathogens, while increased hospital stays put elderly patients at more risk for exposure to hospital-acquired infections (nosocomial infections). Appropriate body substance isolation (BSI) and PPE precautions should be taken to prevent the spread of infection both to and from geriatric patients.

Critical Thinking Question

In addition to having a weak immune response, what else puts an older patient at risk of severe illness due to infection?

Genitourinary System

Kidney filtration function decreases progressively from ages 20 to 90, up to approximately 50%. With decreased filtration function, toxins, such as medications, are not excreted as readily by the renal system. Aging kidneys also respond less efficiently to stress due to decreased blood flow and degeneration of the tubules, which can cause hemodynamic stress as well as fluid and electrolyte imbalances (**FIGURE 1-9**).

Urinary output is also affected. Prostate hypertrophy in men can cause an increased urge to urinate, though the output is minimal. Diminished bladder capacity in both men and women also reduces urinary output. Urinary retention due to prostate enlargement

Renal Function Decline

By the age of 90 years, the mass of the kidneys will decline by 20%, and 50% of filtration function will be lost.

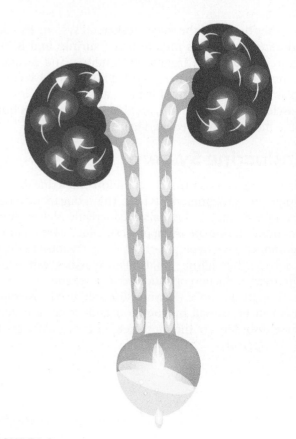

FIGURE 1-9 Kidney function; arrows indicate the direction of flow.
© TimeLineArtist/Shutterstock

in men, and incontinence and nocturnal voiding in men and women due to urinary sphincter dysfunction are common problems.

Critical Thinking Question

Why does deteriorating kidney function put elderly patients at greater risk for drug interaction problems?

Mental Health (Psychological)

Depression, anxiety, and **adjustment disorders** are the most common psychological problems affecting older adults. These conditions can arise organically, result from life situations like social isolation, or be associated with medication use or medical conditions, such as heart disease or diabetes mellitus.

Note that cognitive decline is *not* a normal part of aging. The presence of any cognitive decline (e.g., dementia) is a result of other factors, either or both pathologic or lifestyle (**FIGURE 1-10**).

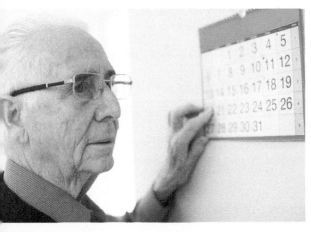

FIGURE 1-10 Many factors contribute to decline in cognitive function in older adults.

aisy Daisy/Shutterstock

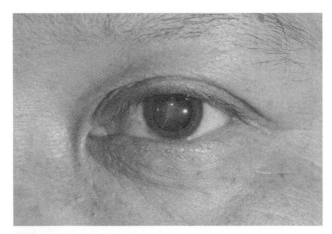

FIGURE 1-11 Cataract.

© ARZTSAMUI/Shutterstock

Lead with Active Listening, Empathy, and Patience

Older adults often endure medical illness, physical limitations, and social loss all at the same time—a frustrating and stressful combination that can lead to demanding or controlling behavior by the patient. To avoid frustration with the patient if you encounter resistance or other difficult behaviors, take a moment to remember the extreme psychosocial stress this demographic suffers daily, and that these are not personal attacks.

Critical Thinking Question

Can you think of life situations that may cause an older patient to suffer conditions such as depression, anxiety, or adjustment disorders?

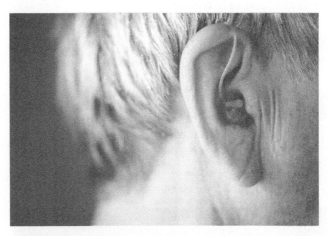

FIGURE 1-12 Modern hearing aid.

© edwardolive/Shutterstock

Many older adults require hearing aids (**FIGURE 1-12**), although they do not always get them, which can lead to additional problems such as isolation and depression.

Communication Is Key

If a patient uses a hearing aid, keep it in place (if possible) to allow for better communication and assessment both during your initial assessment and for transport to the hospital, so the patient may effectively communicate with personnel there as care continues.

Sensory Changes

ensory changes occur to an older person's vision and earing. Optic changes include smaller pupils, development of cataracts (**FIGURE 1-11**) and lens thickening eading to blurring of vision), and decreased ability to ee at night. Eye exams in the field may produce a limed upward gaze in the patient due to degenerative hanges in the eyes' elevator muscles.

Hearing loss is four times more common than vision npairment, with high-frequency hearing lost first. hanges to the structure of the ear can lead to deafness.

Barriers to Care

Older patients may present challenges for the EMS practitioner in assessment and treatment due to physical and cognitive changes associated with the aging process. These changes, referred to as **barriers to care**, can affect behavior and ability to effectively communicate what is happening. These same factors may also cause older persons to avoid seeking medical care.

Barriers to care include:

- Hearing difficulty
- Poor vision
- Decreased mobility (most commonly reported; an estimated 1 in 4 patients experience decreased mobility)
- Difficulty with decision making
- Poor memory recall
- Difficulty concentrating
- Inability to independently perform activities of daily living, such as bathing, dressing, and preparing meals
- Fear of loss of independence

Older patients might refuse care due to loss of their independence or fear of being admitted to a hospital or sent to a nursing home.

Unequal Barriers

Barriers to care affect women more often than men. Poverty increases these barriers for all older persons.

Critical Thinking Question

How do barriers to care impede patient assessment and treatment, and what strategies should you use to overcome them?

The GEMS Diamond

The GEMS Diamond acronym was created to remind the EMS practitioner how geriatric patients differ from younger patient groups. It is not intended to be a format for the approach to assessing a geriatric patient; rather, it should be integrated throughout the assessment to create a complete picture of any special considerations for the patient (**FIGURE 1-13**). The GEMS Diamond augments the assessment approach you normally use by reminding you of additional assessment points that may not be as relevant for a younger patient.

G for Geriatric Assessment

The geriatric age group will present with medical conditions and emergencies differently than younger patients. For example, what may be a minor fall for a

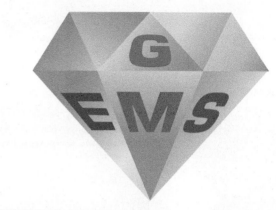

FIGURE 1-13 GEMS Diamond.
© Jones & Bartlett Learning

young patient can cause serious injury to the geriatric patient. Improvement in emergency care of older persons occurs when EMS practitioners have increased knowledge of the physical and psychosocial issues facing the older population, feel confident communicating with them, and understand the management and care of injured older adults. For example, extra questions may be required if the patient is confused; or, if the patient has hearing loss, speaking louder and enunciating while facing the patient can help increase efficiency in your assessment.

E for Environment Assessment

A patient's environment can reveal clues to the root cause of the emergency (or related comorbidities). Assess the patient's living condition for safety and hygiene, maintenance, hazardous conditions, temperature (too hot or cold?), and evidence of difficulty performing acts of daily living, such as preparing meals and going to the toilet. Aging changes can be subtle and caregivers as well as patients may not notice them or may normalize living conditions that have gradually deteriorated to the point of potential risk to the patient's well-being.

M for Medical Assessment

The older patient typically has several medical problems and may be taking various prescription or over-the-counter medications. Obtaining a thorough medical history is essential for all patients, including those with traumatic injury.

S for Social Assessment

Assess the older patient for the level of social support available as well as evidence of neglect and abuse. Look for signs of depression and anxiety, which can be

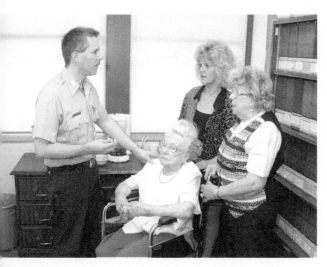

FIGURE 1-14 Assess the patient's social network to determine level of available social support.
© Jack Hollingsworth/Photodisc/Getty Images

caused by a shrinking social network, loss of friends or a spouse, and separation from family. Assess if the patient needs assistance to perform activities of daily living (**FIGURE 1-14**).

> ### Support Social and Emotional Well-Being
>
> Consider if the patient has sufficient social support for both their physical and emotional needs.

Assessment Pathway

Following a systematic assessment approach whenever initial patient contact is made provides a safe and efficient patient evaluation. While the geriatric patient assessment follows the same approach as for younger adults, there are additional considerations, as suggested by the GEMS Diamond. These include:

- Geriatric patients tend to have more complexity to their medical condition and present differently compared to younger patients.
- A patient's clinical presentation could include a variety of unexpected symptoms.
- Assessing quality of life and functional status is necessary when evaluating the patient's independence.
- Limited mobility and possible frailty may reduce the ability of the patient to maintain their health.

Assessment principles should include the chief complaint, primary survey, chronic conditions, review of medication list, polypharmacy categorization, and mental and physical status.

> ### Same Assessment Goals for All Patients
>
> - Find and treat any life threats.
> - Determine the priority of care.

Scene Size-Up

As with all calls, patient assessment begins with scene size-up. Once you have addressed personal safety concerns, gain access to the patient and assess the environment for any clues to their medical condition or cause of complaint. When dealing with a trauma incident, assess for mechanism of injury while recalling that much less force is required to cause injury to a geriatric patient.

While approaching the patient, rapidly assess the patient's level of distress. The general impression should be a rapid global overview of the status of a patient's respiratory, circulatory, and neurologic systems. Observe if the patient is alert and interactive or not, the level of work of breathing, and the appearance of the skin for adequacy of perfusion.

> ### Just Looking
>
> The scene size-up involves no physical contact with the patient.

Primary Survey

The primary survey is a limited physical assessment intended to identify any immediate life threats (**TABLE 1-1**). The assessment process investigates the most immediate life-threatening cause to the least. This process is interrupted only to manage a life threat when identified, and the assessment is resumed once the life threat has been addressed. The primary survey should follow the XABCDE approach.

Secondary Assessment

Following the primary survey (XABCDE), practitioners should assess vital signs, including obtaining a 12-lead ECG tracing, conduct history taking using the OPQRST and SAMPLER mnemonics, and perform a more detailed physical exam. Note that obtaining historical information before performing a physical exam is dependent on the patient's initial presentation.

Ongoing Assessment

The patient should be assessed repeatedly to determine response to EMS interventions and to otherwise

TABLE 1-1 Primary Survey

Primary Survey	
X (exsanguinating hemorrhage)	Assess for severe external bleeding
A (airway)	Assess the airway for patency and risk for obstruction; consider need for spinal motion restriction, recalling that a much lower threshold for injury is required for geriatric patients
B (breathing)	Assess breathing adequacy and potential for deterioration
C (circulation)	Estimate blood pressure by palpating pulse points; assess the skin for color, warmth, and moisture
D (disability)	Calculate Glasgow Coma Scale (GCS) score, and assess pupil equality and light response
E (expose/ environment)	Brief but thorough assessment of the patient's body for any significant injury or medical condition; consider risk of body heat loss prior to exposing the patient and cover or reclothe as soon as possible

Copyright © 2024 National Association of Emergency Medical Technicians (NAEMT).

monitor the patient while in EMS care. The ongoing assessment can be considered in four steps:

1. Repetition of the initial assessment: Repeat every 15 minutes for a stable patient and every 5 minutes for an unstable patient.
2. Repetition of the vital signs assessment after the initial assessment. This secondary survey step identifies trends of improvement or deterioration in the patient.
3. Repetition of the focused assessment. You may need to repeat important steps of the detailed physical exam.
4. Evaluation of the patient's response to medical interventions that have been provided.

Do Not Ignore Your Patient

Geriatric patients can deteriorate suddenly and without warning!

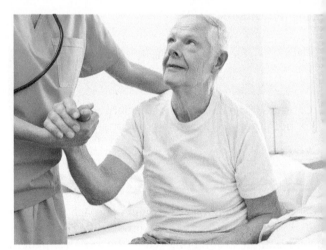

FIGURE 1-15 Immobility problems may prevent older adults from moving well or safely. Performing the 'Get Up and Go' test can help you assess the level of immobility in your patient.
© Robert Kneschke/Shutterstock

Five Is

The 'Five Is' is another memory aid that is helpful when assessing and caring for a geriatric patient. This aid provides a reminder for disorders common in the geriatric patient population (**FIGURE 1-15**).

Rapid Geriatric Assessment

Developed at Saint Louis University, the Rapid Geriatric Assessment includes four screening tools and confirmation of an advance care directive to assist practitioners in identifying a geriatric patient's syndrome.

1. FRAIL scale
2. SARC-F scale
3. Rapid cognitive screen (RCS)
4. Simplified nutritional assessment questionnaire (SNAQ65+)

The Five Is

1. **I**ntellectual impairment: is the patient alert and attentive; is the patient confused and to what degree?
2. **I**mmobility: steadiness of gait and balance; use the 'Get Up and Go' test, which involves having the patient repeatedly get up from a seated position and walk a short distance.
3. **I**nstability: assess for frailty, failure to thrive, evidence of malnutrition and unplanned weight loss, dehydration, and muscle wasting.
4. **I**ncontinence: assess for presence; use the DIAPPERS mnemonic to consider causes of incontinence in the geriatric patient.
   - **D**elirium, **I**nfection, **A**trophic urethritis, **P**harmacy-induced, **P**sychological, **E**xcess urinary output, **R**estricted mobility, and **S**tool impaction
5. **I**atrogenic disorder: consider if current complaint is related to adverse reaction to medication or interactions between medications.

CHAPTER WRAP-UP

- The proportion of those aged older than 65 years is increasing.
- Every body system is negatively impacted by the aging process, causing many older patients to have multiple medical conditions and more complex medical histories than younger patients.
- Using the GEMS Diamond as part of the assessment pathway for older patients will help identify geriatric-specific concerns and improve the effectiveness of assessments.
- Ongoing assessments are necessary to effectively monitor the older patient for changes.

- Remember the four considerations when assessing a geriatric patient:
  1. They tend to have more complex issues than a young adult.
  2. Evaluating the quality of life and functional status is an essential part of determining their independence.
  3. Their frailty level determines the physiologic ability to maintain homeostasis.
  4. Assessment principles should include the chief complaint, chronic conditions, review of medication list, polypharmacy categorization, and mental and physical status.

REFERENCES

Alshibani A, Alharbi M, Conroy S. Under-triage of older trauma patients in prehospital care: a systematic review. *Eur Geriatr Med*. 2021 Oct;12(5):903–919. doi:10.1007/s41999-021-00512-5

America Counts Staff. *2020 Census Will Help Policymakers Prepare for the Incoming Wave of Aging Boomers*. United States Census Bureau. https://www.census.gov/library/stories/2019/12/by-2030-all-baby-boomers-will-be-age-65-or-older.html#:~:text=In%202018%2C%20there%20were%2052. Accessed April 2, 2022.

Azimi I, Rahmani AM, Liljeberg P, et al. Internet of things for remote elderly monitoring: a study from user-centered perspective. *J Ambient Intell Humaniz Comput*. 2017;8(2):273–289.

Centers for Disease Control and Prevention. *Prevalence of Disabilities and Health Care*. https://www.cdc.gov/ncbddd/disabilityand health/features/kf-adult-prevalence-disaiblities.html. Published November 2018. Accessed April 6, 2022.

Chu I, Vaca F, Stratton S, et al. Geriatric trauma care: challenges facing emergency medical services. *Cal J Emerg Med*. 2007 May;8(2):51–55.

Dickinson ET, Verdile VP, Kostyun CT, Salluzzo RF. Geriatric use of emergency medical services. *Ann Emerg Med*. 1996 Feb;27(2):199–203.

Fuentes E, Fuentes M, Alarcón M, Palomo I. Immune system dysfunction in the elderly. *An Acad Bras Cienc*. 2017 Jan–Mar;89(1):285–299.

Gregg EW, Engelgau MM, Narayan V. Complications of diabetes in elderly people. *BMJ*. 2002 Oct;325(7370):916–917.

He W, et al. *An Aging World: 2015*. Washington, DC: United States Census Bureau; 2015.

Jones CMC, Wasserman EB, Li T, Amidon A, Abbott M, Shah MN. The effect of older age on EMS use for transportation to an emergency department. *Prehosp Disaster Med*. 2017;32(3):261–268.

Karavidas A, Lazaros G, Tsiachris D, Pyrgakis V. Aging and the cardiovascular system. *Hellenic J Cardiol*. 2010 Sep–Oct;51(5):421–427.

Levitzy MG. Effects of aging on the respiratory system. *Physiologist*. 1984;27(2):102–107.

Park JM, Sohn A. Predictors affecting the elderly's use of emergency medical services. *Osong Public Health Res Perspect*. 2020 Aug;11(4):209–215.

Peterson LK, Fairbanks RJ, Hettinger AZ, Shah MN. Emergency medical service attitudes toward geriatric prehospital care and continuing medical education in geriatrics. *J Am Geriatr Soc*. 2009 Mar;57(3):530–535. doi:10.1111/j.1532-5415.2008.02108.x

Rogers A, Rogers F, Bradburn E, et al. Old and undertriaged: a lethal combination. *Am Surg*. 2012;78(6):711–715. doi:10.1177/000313481207800628

Rosen CJ. Endocrine disorders and osteoporosis. *Curr Opin Rheumatol*. 1997 Jul;9(4):355–361. doi:10.1097/00002281-199707000-00014

Rosso A, Studenski S, Chen W, et al. Aging, the central nervous system, and mobility. *J Gerontol A Biol Sci Med Sci*. 2013 Nov;68(11):1379–1386. doi:10.1093/gerona/glt089

Rural Health Information Hub. *Demographic Changes and Aging Population*. https://www.ruralhealthinfo.org/toolkits/aging/1/demographics. Last reviewed June 4, 2019. Accessed on April 2, 2022.

Saint Louis University School of Medicine. Assessments, Tools, and Resources. https://www.slu.edu/medicine/internal-medicine/geriatric-medicine/aging-successfully/assessment-tools/index.php. Accessed April 25, 2022.

Shah MN, Bazarian JJ, Lerner EB, et al. The epidemiology of emergency medical services use by older adults: an analysis of the National Hospital Ambulatory Medical Care Survey. *Acad Emerg Med*. 2007 May;14(5):441–447. doi:10.1197/j.aem.2007.01.019

Sözen T, Özışık L, Başaran NÇ. An overview and management of osteoporosis. *Eur J Rheumatol*. 2017;4(1):46–56. doi:10.5152/eurjrheum.2016.048

Tosato M, Zamboni V, Ferrini A, Cesari M. The aging process and potential interventions to extend life expectancy. *Clin Interv Aging*. 2007;2(3):401–412.

Trunkey DD, Cahn RM, Lenfesty B, Mullins R. Management of the geriatric trauma patient at risk of death: therapy withdrawal decision making. *Arch Surg*. 2000;135(1):34–38. doi:10.1001/archsurg.135.1.34

United Nations. Shifting demographics. https://www.un.org/en/un75/shifting-demographics#:~:text=Older%20persons%20(ages%2065%20and,(ages%2015%20to%2024). Accessed August 28, 2022.

United States Census Bureau. *2017 National Population Projections Tables: Main Series*. https://www.census.gov/data/tables/2017/demo/popproj/2017-summary-tables.html. Accessed on April 2, 2022.

World Health Organization. *Healthy Ageing and Functional Ability*. https://www.who.int/news-room/questions-and-answers/item/healthy-ageing-and-functional-ability. Published October 26, 2020. Accessed April 25, 2022.

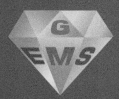

CHAPTER 2

Polypharmacy and Toxicity in Older Patients

LESSON OBJECTIVES

- Define polypharmacy, specifically as it applies to the geriatric patient population.
- Demonstrate the assessment of and link between polypharmacy and toxicity.
- Differentiate between pharmacokinetics and pharmacodynamics.

- Recognize the effects of medication noncompliance, dosing errors, and toxidromes in older patients.
- Discuss management of polypharmacy, medication noncompliance, and toxicity in geriatric patients.

Introduction

Polypharmacy is usually defined as regularly using multiple medications concurrently (**FIGURE 2-1**). Some patients may take up to 21 prescription medications daily. Because older adults are living longer with chronic medical conditions and respond differently to medications when compared with younger patients, geriatric patients have an increased risk of adverse reactions. The potential for both intentional and unintentional issues with medication compliance also increases with the number of drugs prescribed.

Prescription Noncompliance

Prescription noncompliance is estimated to be 79% for medications taken once daily. Noncompliance reduces to approximately 51% when the drug is to be taken four times per day.

Polypharmacy and Adverse Drug Events

The American Geriatric Society (AGS) recognized the dangers of inappropriate medication prescriptions and the associated adverse drug events, or medicine-induced

harm, resulting from them. In 2011, the AGS adopted the Beers Criteria® for Potentially Inappropriate Medication Use in Older Adults. The criteria are updated every 3 years, most recently in 2019.

The AGS Beers Criteria® includes five lists describing medications that should be:

1. Avoided by most older people (outside of hospice and palliative care settings)
2. Avoided by older people with specific health conditions
3. Avoided in combination with other treatments due to the risk for harmful "drug–drug" interactions
4. Used with caution due to *potential* for harmful side effects
5. Dosed differently or avoided in people with reduced kidney function (which impacts how the body processes medicine)

Polypharmacy is necessary for care of older patients with multiple medical conditions, and even with the Beers Criteria® available to guide prescribers, it increases the complexity of organizing and administering the medications. Omitting, overdosing, and mistiming errors in drug administration are common.

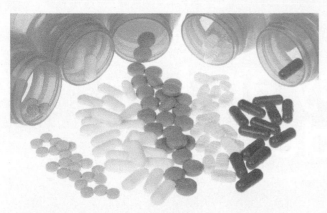

FIGURE 2-1 Older adults are often prescribed multiple medications, leading to the potential for adverse reactions.
© Sheila Fitzgerald/Shutterstock

That's a Lot of Pills

According to the CDC's National Center for Health Statistics, more than 90% of older persons use at least one medication, and more than 66% use three or more.

Polypharmacy also increases the risk of experiencing an **adverse drug event (ADE)**. An ADE occurs when a patient is harmed by a drug. This result is due to one drug interacting with another drug or a drug reacting to a disease or organ dysfunction. Research indicates that patients taking more than two medications have an increased risk of an ADE, and patients taking more than seven medications have an 82% chance of an ADE.

Drug Inequity

Females are 1.5 times more likely to experience an ADE than are males. There are sex-based differences suspected to be part of the cause; however, how these differences result in an increased ADE risk is unclear:

- Sex-related differences in pharmacokinetic, immunologic, and hormonal factors
- Differences in the types of medications used by females compared with males
- Females have lower lean body mass compared to males
- Females have reduced hepatic clearance compared to males

Critical Thinking Question

How does polypharmacy complicate emergency medical assessment in the older adult?

Medication Toxicity

Medication toxicity in older adults can result from overdose; or it can occur from a gradual accumulation of medication in the bloodstream due to dosing error; changes in enzymatic activity, which alter rates of drug metabolism; and reduced excretion by impaired kidney, liver, or lung function. Effects of medication toxicity in a geriatric patient include the following:

- Direct effect on the medication's target organ
- Collateral damage to the lungs or renal system
- Immunosuppression, increasing risk of infection; or, enhanced immune response that can worsen autoimmune disorders

Medication toxicity can also result as a factor of age-related changes to the drug pharmacokinetics. Absorption of the drug into the bloodstream is reduced by changes in the gastrointestinal (GI) tract, inhibiting the medication dissolving and being absorbed in the mucosa. However, decreased GI tract motility leads to higher blood levels of the drug. Distribution is affected by the increased fat tissue and decrease in plasma proteins. These two changes increase the availability of the drug in circulation.

Pharmacokinetics & Pharmacodynamics

Pharmacokinetics is often confused with **pharmacodynamics**. Pharmacokinetics describes what the body does to the administered drug. This dynamic is affected by the aging process. Pharmacodynamics describes what the administered drug does to the body. It is unclear whether or how pharmacodynamics is affected by the aging process (**TABLE 2-1**).

Drug metabolism slows due to aging changes in the liver. First pass effect through the liver is reduced, so

TABLE 2-1 Pharmacokinetics versus Pharmacodynamics	
Pharmacokinetics	**Pharmacodynamics**
What the *body* does to the administered *drug*	What the administered *drug* does to the *body*
Body → Drug	Drug → Body
Affected by the aging process	Unclear if affected by the aging process

fewer drug metabolites are produced, and drug levels in the bloodstream are higher than for a younger patient. Similarly, age-related changes to the kidneys reduce the rate of elimination of the drug and its metabolites from the bloodstream.

Drug toxicity can impact older patients in the following ways:

- *Distribution:* Movement of the drug to and from blood and tissue changes as lean muscle mass declines and fat percentage increases. A decrease in the amount of plasma proteins leads to an increase in the availability of the drug in circulation. A normal dose in a younger patient could prove to be toxic in a geriatric patient.
- *Metabolism* (detoxification): The liver is the primary site for drug metabolism. A group of enzymes known as cytochrome P-450 enzymes are responsible for drug metabolism, and the availability of these enzymes decreases with age. Reductions in these enzymes may affect metabolism of the drug, causing drug levels to rise, increasing both the effects and side effects of the drug. As the liver becomes less effective at removing the medication there is also a greater risk of drug–drug interaction or a single drug toxicity.
- *Absorption:* Drugs taken orally are more poorly dissolved and absorbed in the GI tract of geriatric patients due to aging mucosa and a decrease in gastric acid and digestive enzyme production, leading to changes in intestinal motility. However, the decline in stomach motility allows more time for a drug to be absorbed into the bloodstream, leading to higher-than-normal levels of the drug.
- *Elimination:* As the kidneys lose their ability to filter and eliminate drugs there can be an accumulation of drugs in the blood, leading to the potential for a toxic effect.

Common conditions that could increase the likelihood of drug toxicity in the geriatric cohort include diabetes, heart disease, hypertension, renal failure, chronic obstructive pulmonary disease, and malnutrition.

- Medications for controlling high blood sugar levels (e.g., insulin) can cause dangerously high or low blood sugar levels.
- Medications for controlling cardiac rate and function (e.g., beta blockers, calcium channel blockers) can cause dysrhythmias.
- Medications for managing high blood pressure (e.g., angiotensin-converting enzyme [ACE] inhibitors, angiotensin receptor blockers [ARBs]) can lead to low blood pressure.
- Medications for controlling body fluid levels (e.g., nonpotassium-sparing diuretics) can lead to electrolyte abnormality such as hypokalemia.

- Medications for managing chronic obstructive pulmonary disease (e.g., bronchodilators, anticholinergics, steroids) can lead to anticholinergic symptoms, such as bladder incontinence.
- Malnutrition may lead to low serum protein and dehydration, which can affect concentrations of medications in the bloodstream.

Toxidrome Presentation in the Geriatric Population

Due to the complexity of a geriatric patient's medical history and health status, cases of acute poisoning involving this age group can be challenging to identify and manage. A **toxidrome** is the constellation of signs and symptoms caused by a class of toxin. Recognition of a toxidrome can help diagnose the type of toxin involved and indicate the appropriate antidote.

Sympathomimetic Toxidrome

Agents causing a sympathomimetic toxidrome include caffeine, nicotine, cocaine, and theophylline. Signs that may be found include hypertension, tachycardia, tachypnea, hyperthermia, agitation, and dilated pupils.

Cholinergic Toxidrome

Agents in the cholinergic toxidrome group include insecticides, nicotine, pilocarpine, and bethanechol chloride. Two memory aids are often used to remind clinicians of the effects of this toxidrome:

1. SLUDGEM: **S**alivation, **L**acrimation, **U**rination, **D**efecation, **G**astrointestinal upset, **E**mesis, and **M**uscle twitching/**M**iosis (pupillary constriction)
2. DUMBBELS: **D**iarrhea, **U**rination, **M**iosis, **B**ronchorrhea/**B**ronchoconstriction, **B**radycardia, **E**mesis, **L**acrimation, and **S**alivation/**S**weating

Anticholinergic Toxidrome

Agents that may cause an anticholinergic toxidrome include antihistamines, tricyclic antidepressants, atropine, cyclobenzaprine, and antiparkinsonian agents. Effects of this toxidrome include agitated delirium (often with hallucinations, incoherent speech, picking at the air or objects), flushed skin, dry skin (check armpits for lack of sweat), hyperthermia, pupillary dilation causing blurry vision and photophobia, and urinary retention and reduced bowel sounds. Severe cases may involve seizure and/or coma.

To remember the effects of anticholinergic toxidrome, use the phrase, *"Mad as a hatter, red as a beet, dry as a bone, hot as a hare, blind as a bat, and full as a flask."*

Narcotic/Opioid Toxidrome

Narcotic medications are commonly used to provide pain relief and include codeine, oxycodone (**FIGURE 2-2**), hydrocodone, tramadol, and fentanyl. This class of drug overdose will cause altered mental status, respiratory depression, pinpoint pupils, and somnolence.

Sedative-Hypnotic Toxidrome

A sedative-hypnotic toxidrome may be caused by benzodiazepines, barbiturates, and zolpidem. Presentation of this toxidrome may involve respiratory depression, ataxia, blurred vision, coma, confusion, delirium, diplopia, hallucinations, nystagmus, paresthesia, sedation, slurred speech, and stupor.

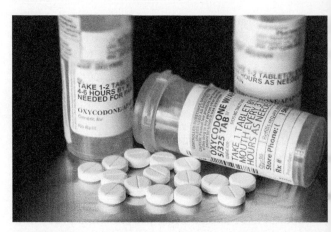

FIGURE 2-2 Oxycodone is a commonly prescribed narcotic for pain.
© Steve Heap/Shutterstock

CASE STUDY

You and your partner are staffing an emergency response ambulance in a suburban neighborhood. You are dispatched to a residence for an unresponsive 78-year-old female (**FIGURE 2-3**).

QUESTIONS

- What conditions are on your differential diagnosis list?
  - Stroke
  - TBI
  - Toxicity
  - Arrhythmia
  - Liver failure
  - Diabetic emergency
  - Electrolyte imbalance
  - UTI
  - Sepsis

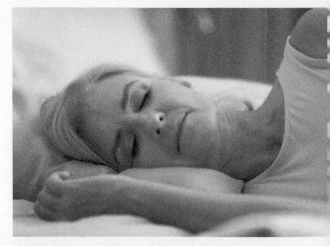

FIGURE 2-3 Patient is an unresponsive 78-year-old female.
© fizkes/Shutterstock

- How does the patient's age affect your assessment approach?
  - Given the patient's age, you will include the GEMS Diamond elements in your assessment (refer to Lesson 1).

As you arrive at the front entrance of the home, you are met by the patient's frail husband (**FIGURE 2-4**). You enter the home and note the living conditions. The home is well-kept, there are no odors, and it appears safe to enter. The temperature in the house is warm. The husband leads you to the patient who is lying in bed. She is appropriately dressed and appears to have proper nutrition for her age. She appears unresponsive. The husband tells you that his wife is rarely ill. They receive meals from a community service three times a week; but otherwise, his wife prepares meals and is his primary caretaker. Their grown children live far away and call occasionally to check on them.

The husband tells you that his wife took her medication last night, as she usually does before going to bed. She slept in longer than usual today and her husband called 911 when he couldn't wake her.

The primary survey reveals the following:

- X–No obvious external bleeding noted
- A–Patent with occasional snoring respirations
- B–Respirations are regular, deep, and slow. Lung sounds are clear and equal bilaterally.
- C–Radial pulses are regular, rapid, and weak. Capillary refill time is 4 seconds. Skin is pale, cool, and moist.
- D–Responsive only to painful stimuli, GCS 8 (E2, V2, M4)
- E–Lying in bed; no further injuries or signs of trauma found on exposure

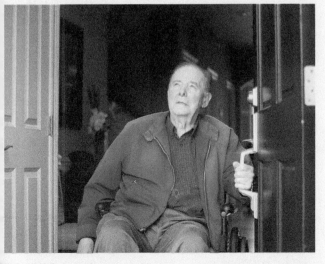

FIGURE 2-4 The patient's husband greets you and leads you to his wife.
© Jaren Jai Wicklund/Shutterstock

QUESTIONS

- What is the cardinal presentation and the chief complaint?
  - Cardinal presentation (what you see): Unresponsive
  - Chief complaint (what the patient reports): Cannot be determined because the patient is not responsive
- Does this patient require immediate transport, or can you remain on scene and continue assessing?
  - Although there is potential for airway compromise (suggested by snoring respirations) and altered mental status, you should continue your assessment on scene.
- What does your list of differential diagnoses include now?
  - Stroke
  - TBI
  - Toxicity
  - Liver failure
  - Diabetic emergency
  - Electrolyte imbalance
  - UTI
  - Sepsis
- What further assessments should you perform?
  - OPQRST, SAMPLER, vital signs, blood glucose test, cardiac monitor, oximeter, detailed physical assessment

You use the OPQRST mnemonic (**o**nset, **p**rovocation, **q**uality, **r**adiation/**r**egion, **s**everity, and **t**ime) to assess the characteristics of the patient's symptoms, but it does not yield any information in this case—all are "unknown."

- O–Unknown
- P–Unknown
- Q–Unknown
- R–Unknown
- S–Unknown
- T–Unknown

You elicit the history of the cardinal presentation as best you can using the SAMPLER mnemonic (**s**igns and symptoms, **a**llergies, **m**edications, **p**ertinent medical history, **l**ast oral intake, **e**vents preceding, **r**isk factors). The husband tells you she took 45 units of insulin lispro and 16 units of insulin glargine before going to bed after assessing her blood glucose level to be > 300 mg/dl (> 16.7 mmol/l). He estimates she went to bed at 2100 hours.

- S–Altered mental status; deep, slow breathing; weak radial pulse; pale, cool, moist skin
- A–No known drug allergies
- M–Metformin, clopidogrel, nitroglycerin tabs, metoprolol, insulin lispro, insulin glargine
- P–Diabetes, angina, CABG 1 vessel (2 years ago)

- L–Snack before bed (toast and herbal tea)
- E–The patient was found with AMS 15 minutes ago by her husband
- R–Age, diabetes, cardiac conditions

The patient's husband tells you that the patient has no drug allergies, and she is compliant with her prescriptions of metformin, clopidogrel, nitroglycerin, metoprolol, insulin lispro, and insulin glargine. Her medical history is diabetes mellitus, angina, and a coronary artery bypass graft (CABG) of one vessel 2 years ago. She has been eating normally and had toast and herbal tea before going to bed. The patient's husband does not recall any unusual events before he found her unresponsive 15 minutes prior to your arrival.

QUESTION

- Review the patient's medication list. Given the polypharmacy, what is the potential for mixing up medications?
  - This patient is on three different medications used to manage diabetes mellitus, which increases the risk of incorrect dosing and/or drug interactions.

In your initial treatment, you position the patient to allow drainage of the airway, and oxygen is provided at 3 lpm by nasal cannula.

You further assess the patient by checking her vital signs, performing a blood glucose test, and attaching a cardiac monitor and oximeter to her. The results of these assessments are:

- HR: 110, regular
- SpO$_2$: 94% on room air
- ETCO$_2$: 43 mm Hg
- RR: 10
- BP: 136/86
- Temp: 97.6°F (36.4°C)
- ETCO$_2$ Waveform: Normal boxed
- 4-lead ECG: Sinus tachycardia
- BGL: 12 mg/dl (0.67 mmol/l)

QUESTION

- What do these vital signs tell you about this patient?
  - The patient is hypoglycemic.
  - Heart rate is high and respirations are slow, which could be caused by hypoglycemia.

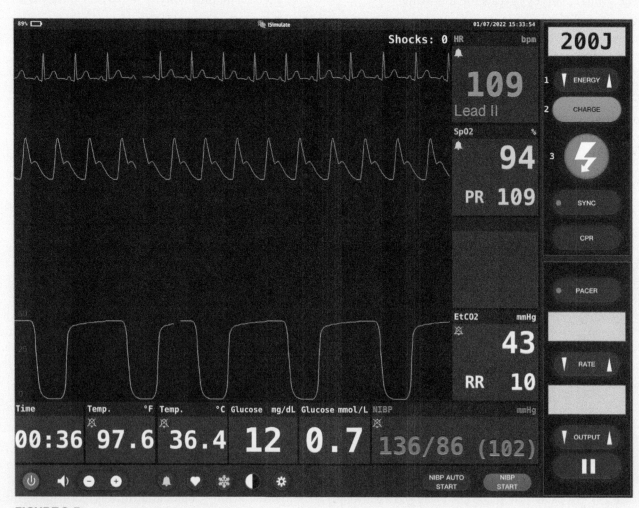

FIGURE 2-5

A 12-lead ECG shows sinus tachycardia.
A detailed physical assessment reveals the following:

- HEENT
  - Head–Unremarkable
  - Eyes–Pupils midpoint and reactive
  - Ears–Unremarkable
  - Nose–Unremarkable
  - Throat–Unremarkable

- Heart and Lungs
  - Lung sounds: clear and equal bilaterally
  - Heart sounds: normal without murmur, rubs, or gallops

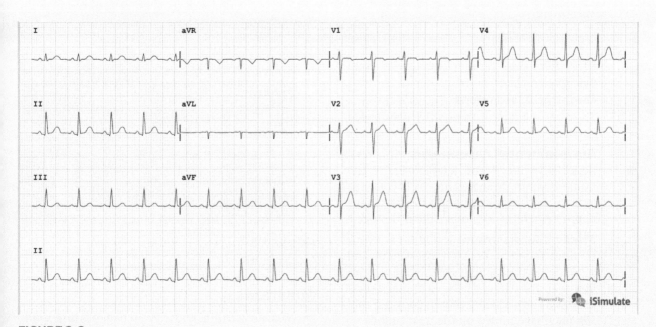

FIGURE 2-6

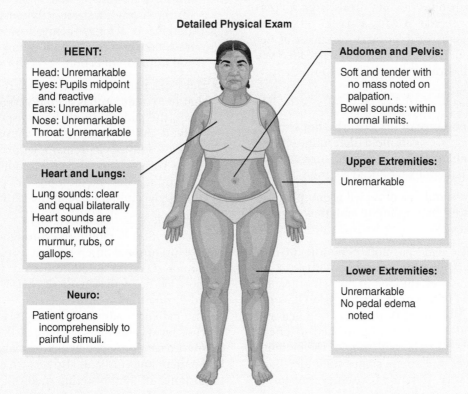

Detailed Physical Exam

HEENT:
Head: Unremarkable
Eyes: Pupils midpoint and reactive
Ears: Unremarkable
Nose: Unremarkable
Throat: Unremarkable

Heart and Lungs:
Lung sounds: clear and equal bilaterally
Heart sounds are normal without murmur, rubs, or gallops.

Neuro:
Patient groans incomprehensibly to painful stimuli.

Abdomen and Pelvis:
Soft and tender with no mass noted on palpation.
Bowel sounds: within normal limits.

Upper Extremities:
Unremarkable

Lower Extremities:
Unremarkable
No pedal edema noted

FIGURE 2-7

- Neuro
  - Patient groans incomprehensibly to painful stimuli.

- Abdomen and Pelvis
  - Soft and tender with no mass noted on palpation
  - Bowel sounds: within normal limits

- Upper Extremities
  - Unremarkable

- Lower Extremities
  - Unremarkable
  - No pedal edema noted

GEMS DIAMOND REVIEW

How was the GEMS Diamond information applied in this case?

 Geriatric Assessment: The patient is a 78-year-old female with expected age-related changes.

 Environmental Assessment: The residence is well-kept and temperature in the house is warm. No odors noted. The patient is dressed appropriately, and appears to have appropriate nutrition for a patient this age.

 Medical Assessment: In addition to your findings from the detailed assessment and vital signs, the patient's husband advises you that his wife has been taking all medications as prescribed, but you consider that she may have mixed up the medications.

 Social Assessment: The patient can accomplish ADLs on her own; she lives with her husband. They get meals from a community service 3 days a week; otherwise, the patient is the primary caretaker of her husband. Their grown children live far away and call occasionally to check in on them.

QUESTIONS

- What is the importance of the ECG rhythm strip?
  - Obtaining an ECG can help determine if the patient's condition is cardiac related; for example, whether the patient experienced a stroke.

- What treatment should be provided prehospitally?
  - Effective airway management and treatment of hypoglycemia

The patient is placed in a position of comfort and provided oxygen and ventilation assistance (**FIGURE 2-8**). An intravenous line is established in her left antecubital fossa (ACF) and IV dextrose is administered as per local protocol. $D_{10}W$ 250 ml IV drip was initiated and administered at 50–100 ml IV and titrated to effect. Shortly after the dextrose administration, the patient's mentation improves and she becomes fully alert, oriented, and cooperative. Her airway patency is restored, and her vital signs also normalized.

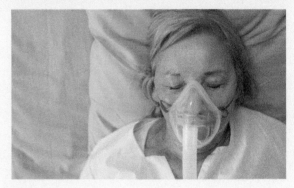

FIGURE 2-8 Oxygen is provided to the patient.
© Ground Picture/Shutterstock

QUESTIONS

- What do you think caused your patient's unresponsive, altered mental status?
  - Hypoglycemia, most likely caused by incorrect dosing of insulin.
  - Insulin lispro is a short-acting insulin, and insulin glargine is a longer-acting insulin. Their dosing must take into consideration their different onsets and duration of action.

- Does this patient require transport to hospital now that her condition has been reversed?
  - Yes, the patient should be transported so that her blood glucose levels can be monitored to ensure they continue to remain within normal range. The patient may also need additional education regarding her medications to prevent another hypoglycemic episode in the future.

The patient is transported to the closest appropriate facility. She is monitored throughout transport to ensure prehospital interventions achieve therapeutic outcomes. Oxygen is administered with ventilatory support via bag-valve mask (BVM). No changes were noted during transport.

The patient is admitted overnight to monitor blood glucose levels and then discharged the next day with follow-up care provided by her primary care physician. The patient and husband also receive education on the importance of administering medication as prescribed to avoid further adverse drug events.

CASE STUDY WRAP-UP

Acute altered mental status is common in the geriatric population; aggressive evaluation and treatment are necessary to prevent a high incidence of mortality. Potential life-threatening causes of acute altered mental status in the geriatric cohort can include infections, polypharmacy, ADEs, dehydration, electrolyte disorders, and intracranial and cardiovascular emergencies.

Insulin prescriptions are available in both fast-acting and long-lasting options. This allows for more balanced control of blood glucose levels. However, this approach requires the patient to dose two versions of the same medication. Occasionally, this dosing can become confused. The resulting error can induce a state of hyper- or hypoglycemia.

Education for the patient and her husband on proper medication usage is imperative.

CHAPTER WRAP-UP

Polypharmacy is prevalent in the geriatric population. Caring for these patients requires an understanding of the importance of assessing the patient's past medical history and all current medications and supplements being taken.

Impaired pharmacokinetics is a normal process of aging that can lead to medication toxicity even when medications are taken as prescribed or directed. Polypharmacy can exacerbate this problem due to unexpected drug interactions.

Toxidromes provide an alternative to learning all drug effects by focusing on the constellation of signs and symptoms related to different classes of drugs. An effective assessment can identify the presence of toxidromes and lead to prompt care.

REFERENCES

American Geriatrics Society. American Geriatrics Society 2015 Updated Beers Criteria for Potentially Inappropriate Medication Use in Older Adults. *J Am Geriatr Soc.* 2015;63(11):2227–2246.

American Geriatrics Society. For Older People, Medications Are Common; Updated AGS Beers Criteria® Aims to Make Sure They're Appropriate, Too. https://www.americangeriatrics.org/media-center/news/older-people-medications-are-common-updated-ags-beers-criteriar-aims-make-sure. Accessed April 25, 2022.

Budnitz DS, Lovegrove MC, Shehab N. Emergency hospitalizations for adverse drug events in older Americans. *N Engl J Med.* 2011;365:2002–2012.

Centers for Disease Control and Prevention. Adverse Drug Events in Adults. https://www.cdc.gov/medicationsafety/adult_adversedrugevents.html. Last reviewed 2017. Accessed April 10, 2022.

Centers for Disease Control and Prevention, National Center for Health Statistics. Table 79: Prescription drug use in the past 30 days, by sex, race and Hispanic origin, and age: United States, selected years 1988–1994 through 2011–2014. https://www.cdc.gov/nchs/data/hus/2017/079.pdf. Accessed April 25, 2022.

Golchin N, Frank SH, Vince A, Isham L, Meropol SB. Polypharmacy in the elderly. *J Res Pharm Pract.* 2015 April–June;4(2):85–88.

Hales CM, Servais J, Martin CB, Kohen D. Prescription Drug Use Among Adults Aged 40–79 in the United States and Canada. Centers for Disease Control and Prevention. https://www.cdc.gov/nchs/products/databriefs/db347.htm. Published 2019. Accessed April 10, 2022.

Lavan AH, Gallagher P. Predicting risk of adverse drug reactions in older adults. *Ther Adv Drug Saf.* 2016;7(1):11–22.

Le J. Drug Metabolism. https://www.merckmanuals.com/home/drugs/administration-and-kinetics-of-drugs/drug-metabolism#:~:text=Most%20drugs%20must%20pass%20through. June 2022. Accessed April 10, 2022.

Maher RL, Hanlon J, Hajjar ER. Clinical consequences of polypharmacy in elderly. *Expert Opin Drug Saf.* 2014;13(1):57–65.

Mattu A. Geriatric emergency medicine. *Emerg Med Clin N Amer.* 2006;24(2):xiii–xiv.

Rehman R, Dawson AH, Hai O. *Digitalis Toxicity.* StatPearls [Internet]. https://www.ncbi.nlm.nih.gov/books/NBK459165/. Updated May 8, 2022. Accessed on April 10, 2022.

Schimpff SC. Normal aging: A steady loss of organ and process function. https://www.kevinmd.com/blog/2017/04/normal-aging-steady-loss-organ-process-function.html#:~:text=Then%20there%20is%20a%20plateau. Published April 20, 2017. Accessed April 10, 2022.

CHAPTER 3

Respiratory Emergencies

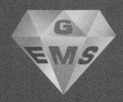

LESSON OBJECTIVES

Discuss the epidemiology, pathophysiology, assessment, and prehospital interventions for older patients with respiratory emergencies.

- Identify the signs and symptoms of a respiratory emergency in a geriatric patient.
- Demonstrate the management of respiratory emergencies.

Introduction

Respiratory disease is a leading cause of death worldwide in older adults. Nearly 1 million people are hospitalized annually for pneumonia, and approximately 90% of pneumonia deaths are in patients older than 65 years.

The respiratory system undergoes significant physiologic and structural changes with aging. These changes are discussed in Chapter 1: Changes with Age. Complicating geriatric clinical presentation further, these aging changes are highly variable from patient to patient. There is no "normal" state for a certain age to use as a baseline for assessing if a disease or disorder is present. The variability of aging effects on the respiratory system may make some patients more susceptible to disease and may explain the differences in response to respiratory therapies.

Influenza: Seasonal Danger

Since 2010, there have been approximately 12,000 to 61,000 deaths per year in the United States due to seasonal influenza virus epidemics. An estimated 90% of seasonal influenza deaths involve geriatric patients.

Respiratory Disease in the Older Adult

Geriatric patients often have comorbidities that share similar signs and symptoms with respiratory disease. Conditions with overlapping symptoms include heart failure, anemia, deconditioning (physiologic changes from immobility for 3 days or longer), conditions causing muscle weakness, and renal disease. Age-related changes to the respiratory physiology (TABLE 3-1) also contribute the loss of reserve capacity, meaning that older adults cannot tolerate periods of respiratory compromise for as long as younger patients.

Critical Thinking Question

Why are symptoms of respiratory disease in the elderly so variable?

One of the first indications of respiratory compromise in an older adult is altered mentation, which can range from anxiety and personality change to confusion or unresponsiveness. The patient or patient's caregiver may also be familiar with current symptoms and relate them to medical conditions the patient has suffered previously. For example, the patient may tell you that their chest feels heavy like it did when they had pneumonia a month ago. Further clues can be found by assessing other comorbidities, medications, recent travel, and recent episodes of cross-contamination or transmission of disease.

TABLE 3-1 Age-Related Respiratory Changes	
Age-Related Changes	**Results**
Airways narrow Loss of airway elasticity Thoracic cage stiffening	Decreased tidal volume, which may make oxygenation more challenging
Kyphosis Scoliosis	Extrapulmonary restriction that may contribute to respiratory compromise Patient positioning more difficult Risk of ventilation-perfusion mismatch
Loss of alveolar wall elasticity	Decrease in gas exchange
Reductions in gas exchange causing a decrease in PaO_2 and increase in CO_2	Decreased sensitivity to hypoxia and hypercapnia so patients are more ill when they feel symptoms
Primary and accessory respiratory muscle loss	Reduced ability to breathe deeply, cough, and expel secretions
Reduced immune system response	Increased risk of infection transmission from another host
Decreased gag and cough reflexes	Increased choking and aspiration risk Increased risk of upper respiratory infection and pneumonia

Copyright © 2024 National Association of Emergency Medical Technicians (NAEMT).

Common Pathologies
SARS-CoV-2 Virus (COVID-19 and Its Variants)

Coronavirus disease 2019 (COVID-19) is a highly infectious disease caused by the SARS-CoV-2 virus. The COVID-19 pandemic disproportionately affected older populations. The pandemic exposed the many disparities of health care, requiring changes in how we treat and respond to older persons' needs, especially in emergency situations.

Patients over age 65 with COVID-19 often present atypically compared to the rest of the population. Instead of breathing problems, fever, and cough, older adults may present with symptoms of functional and even cognitive decline. They may experience loss of appetite, lethargy, falls, and weakness, and may have diarrhea. Confusion, agitation, and fatigue may also be present (**FIGURE 3-1**). Older adults with comorbidities such as diabetes or dementia, tend to have a higher prevalence or intensity of these symptoms. Fever may be absent or lower than in the general population.

According to the Centers for Disease Control and Prevention, older adults are more likely to get very sick from COVID-19 than their younger counterparts. They may require hospitalization, intensive care, or a ventilator, and the risk of death is high. That risk increases for people in their 50s, increases again in adults in their 60s, 70s, and 80s, and adults aged 85 and older are the most likely to get extremely sick.

A vaccine consisting of two shots and boosters is available and recommended for all adults. Additional safety measures are recommended for the vulnerable and during COVID surges, including mask wearing, social distancing, and frequent handwashing.

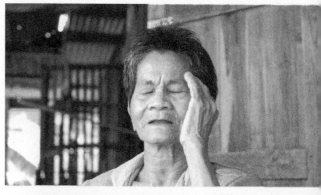

FIGURE 3-1 Older adults suffering a COVID-19 infection may have different symptoms than in the younger population, including confusion, agitation, and even cognitive decline.
© PheungBee Stock/Shutterstock

COVID and the Most Vulnerable Population

As the coronavirus pandemic approached the middle of its third year in 2022, older adults continued to be disproportionately affected. In the United State, 75% of deaths from the coronavirus were in adults 65 years and older. To put that in perspective, for those under age 65, the ratio of deaths to infections was 1 in 1,400. For adults 65 and older, that ratio was 1 death in every 100 cases. As of May 5, 2022, the coronavirus had caused the death of over 15 million people worldwide, according to the World Health Organization.

COVID-19 is currently the third leading cause of death among adults 65 and older, after heart disease and cancer. COVID-19 is responsible for 13% of all deaths in this age group since it was first identified in the United States in the beginning of 2020—more than diabetes, accidents, Alzheimer disease, or other dementias.

Because emergency patient care does not occur in a controlled environment, care and transport of COVID-19 patients by EMS practitioners present unique challenges. Coveralls are an acceptable alternative to gowns when caring for and transporting suspected COVID-19 patients. A fit-tested N95 respirator is recommended for both practitioner and patient, as well as nonsterile disposable gloves and eye protection in areas of high transmission (**FIGURE 3-2**).

Influenza

Influenza is a class of viruses that infects the respiratory tract. The two primary types of influenza are A and B. Influenza infection usually manifests as a contagious and self-limited febrile illness. However, complications of influenza infection can be deadly, especially to those with compromised immune systems or comorbidities, such as with older adults.

Symptom onset is usually sudden and includes cough, sore throat, rhinorrhea, body aches, headache, fatigue, vomiting, diarrhea, and fever (**FIGURE 3-3**). Older adults typically have fewer symptoms and often do not present with a fever. Antiviral medications are commonly prescribed to reduce symptoms and duration of illness.

Prehospital treatment is supportive: empathic care while providing comfort, supplemental oxygen if the patient appears hypoxic, and fluids if signs of dehydration or hypotension are present.

A vaccine is available to prevent the flu and is recommended annually for patients over 65.

Pneumonia

Pneumonia is a viral or bacterial infection of the alveoli. The most common bacterial cause in the United States is from the *Streptococcus pneumoniae* organism. Influenza and rhinovirus (common cold) are the most common viral causes of pneumonia in the United States. These pathogens initiate an inflammatory immune response that causes the alveoli to fill with fluid and pus.

Geriatric patients are at greater risk for pneumonia for a number of reasons. Risk factors are listed in **TABLE 3-2**.

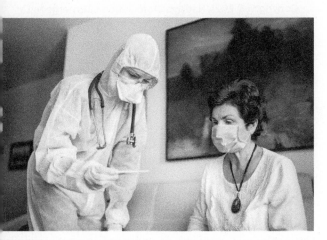

FIGURE 3-2 Because older adults present atypically from younger adults, following your regional protocol for personal protective equipment (PPE) is recommended in all suspected respiratory emergencies.
© eldar nurkovic/Shutterstock

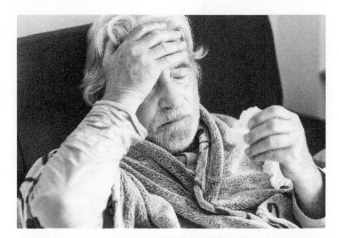

FIGURE 3-3 Influenza can be deadly in older adults and may be harder to recognize as they typically have fewer symptoms and no fever compared to the rest of the population.
© simona pilolla 2/Shutterstock

TABLE 3-2 Risk Factors for Pneumonia

Age-Related Changes	Comorbidities	Other Situations
Weakened immune system response	Chronic obstructive pulmonary disease (COPD)	Hospitalizations
Weakened cough reflex	Diabetes mellitus	Smoking
	Heart failure	Sedation
	Cancer	Ventilator use
	Cerebrovascular accident (CVA; stroke)	Sedentary periods

Copyright © 2024 National Association of Emergency Medical Technicians (NAEMT).

Complications of untreated pneumonia can include:

- Sepsis
- Acute respiratory distress syndrome (ARDS)
- Pleurisy
- Pulmonary abscesses

Symptoms that can occur with pneumonia in the younger adult can occur in the older adult as well. However, the symptoms in older adults are often more subtle than in younger adults (**TABLE 3-3**).

Pneumonia can be subtle and patients may present solely with decreased appetite and increased confusion. Diagnosis is obtained through a medical history, performing a physical examination, and analyzing diagnostics such as blood analysis, chest x-ray, and CT scan.

TABLE 3-3 Signs and Symptoms of Pneumonia Based on Patient Age

Young Adults: Signs and Symptoms	Older Adults: Signs and Symptoms
New or worsening cough	Abnormal lung sounds, such as crackles, wheezes, rhonchi, or locally diminished sounds associated with gradual onset of difficulty breathing
Purulent sputum	
Tachypnea	
Dyspnea	
Tachycardia	Can also present with only decreased appetite and confusion
Pleuritic chest pain	
Fever	Diminished cough reflex leading to less productive cough
Loss of appetite	
Diarrhea	
	Low or no fever

Copyright © 2024 National Association of Emergency Medical Technicians (NAEMT).

Pneumonia: Be Suspicious

Pneumonia should be considered in any geriatric patient exhibiting altered mental status and vague complaints.

Prehospital care is primarily supportive but may include increasing oxygenation and assisting ventilations. Supplemental oxygenation (**FIGURE 3-4**) and bronchodilator therapy may be needed. For patients in severe respiratory distress, consider CPAP and, as a last resort, placement of an advanced airway. Fluid replacement may also be needed if the patient shows signs of dehydration or hypotension.

Ongoing assessment is also more challenging with older patients. End-tidal capnography can be used to monitor the patient and evaluate the patient's response to certain EMS interventions.

A vaccine is available to prevent the most common bacterial cause of pneumonia and is recommended annually for patients over 65.

Chronic Obstructive Pulmonary Disease

Chronic obstructive pulmonary disease (COPD) involves a spectrum of lower airway disease that is chronic and progressive. Conditions associated with COPD include chronic bronchitis, emphysema, and asthma (**FIGURE 3-5**).

Chronic Bronchitis

Chronic bronchitis and emphysema are typically caused by prolonged smoking or exposure to environmental pollutants. Unlike asthma, these two conditions may present together and they are not episodic, but involve ongoing symptoms that can be exacerbated. Exacerbations in the geriatric population are most often due

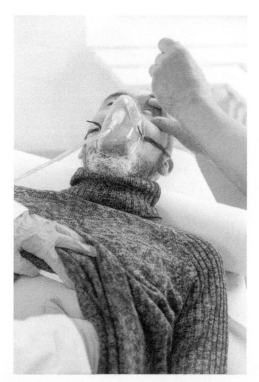

FIGURE 3-4 Supplemental oxygen for patients with pneumonia may be required during prehospital care.
© Miriam Doerr Martin Frommherz/Shutterstock

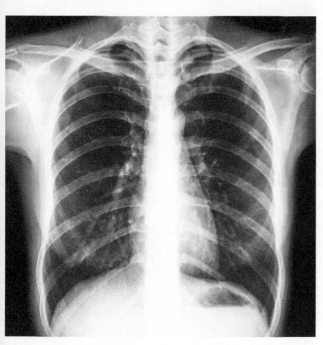

FIGURE 3-5 Radiographic findings of COPD.
© Puwadol Jaturawutthichai/Shutterstock

to infection or poor medication compliance. Chronic bronchitis presents with inflammation of the lower airways and excessive mucus production.

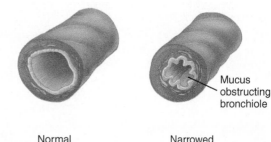

Normal   Narrowed

FIGURE 3-6 Normal and narrowed bronchioles leading to wheezing of asthma.
Copyright © 2024 National Association of Emergency Medical Technicians (NAEMT).

Emphysema

Emphysema involves irreversible destruction of the alveoli and, consequently, air trapping in the chest. Geriatric patients are at increased risk due to comorbid conditions such as dehydration, infection, polypharmacy, and heart disease.

Asthma

Asthma involves episodic spasm of the smooth muscles in the bronchial walls along with edema in the bronchial lining. This occurs in response to exposure to stress, medication, or environmental pollutants. The reactive changes initially lead to expiratory wheezing and progressive air trapping, which causes hyperinflation of the chest, prolonged expiratory phase, and reduced lung sounds.

Clinical Features and Treatment of COPD

Symptoms of an asthma 'attack' or exacerbation of chronic bronchitis or emphysema include increased cough, increased work of breathing, chest tightness, and dyspnea. Signs include gradual onset, possible increased sputum production, accessory muscle use, expiratory wheezing or rhonchi, prolonged expiratory phase, pursed lips to increase PEEP, and right-sided heart failure (**FIGURE 3-6**).

Treatment includes provision of supplemental oxygen and administration of bronchodilators, anticholinergics,

---

Optimizing Gas Exchange

Decreased alveolar elasticity is like a balloon losing its ability to expand. Therefore, decreased alveolar elasticity leads to decreased gas exchange and less oxygen in the blood. A continuous positive airway pressure (CPAP) device can be used to maintain positive end-expiratory pressure (PEEP) to keep the airways and alveoli open and improve gas exchange.

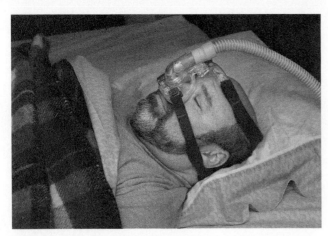

FIGURE 3-7 CPAP ventilatory support.
© Howard Sandler/Shutterstock

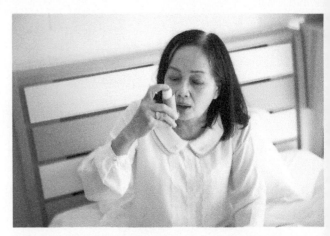

FIGURE 3-8 Bronchodilators are commonly used to treat asthma.
© MISTER DIN/Shutterstock

and steroids. Severe cases will need ventilatory support with continuous positive airway pressure (CPAP) or bi-level positive airway pressure (BiPAP) (**FIGURE 3-7**). Administration of epinephrine and magnesium sulfate may also be required for patients in severe distress.

Asthma and Asthma-COPD Overlap Syndrome

Late-onset asthma can be difficult to differentiate from COPD in older adults. However, both disorders often coexist in older adult patients; this is known as **asthma-COPD overlap syndrome (ACOS**; **FIGURE 3-8**). While asthma alone is a reversible condition, ACOS will worsen over time. The symptoms and management for asthma and ACOS are the same, but the treatment is based on the severity of asthma and COPD. Asthma treatment will focus on suppressing the chronic inflammation, and ACOS treatment will focus on reducing the patient's symptoms.

> ### Treatment Goals
>
> The treatment goal for asthma is to suppress chronic inflammation. The treatment goal for both emphysema and chronic bronchitis is to reduce symptoms.

Acute Bronchitis

Acute bronchitis has the same bronchial irritation and inflammation as chronic bronchitis (**FIGURE 3-9**), but is caused by infection, has rapid onset, and is reversible. This condition is usually caused by viral infection such as influenza, cold, or adenovirus but can also be caused by bacteria. Acute bronchitis typically resolves on its

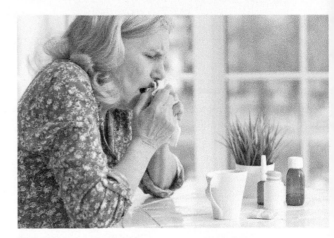

FIGURE 3-9 Irritation and inflammation of the bronchial tubes causes the characteristic coughing of acute bronchitis.
© Ruslan Huzau/Shutterstock

own, but will last longer in geriatric patients. Antibiotics are generally not prescribed, as there is minimal evidence supporting their use as a treatment. Prehospital treatment is therefore primarily supportive.

Acute Respiratory Distress Syndrome

Acute respiratory distress syndrome (ARDS) involves diffuse damage to the lung tissue. Pulmonary inflammation causes increased permeability of the alveolar walls. The increased permeability causes fluid, solutes, and plasma proteins to leak into the alveolar space from the capillaries. As air is displaced from the alveolar space, gas exchange is impaired and respiratory failure occurs.

Common causes include sepsis, inhalation injury due to harmful substances such as smoke or chemicals, aspiration of emesis, and nonfatal drowning.

Signs and symptoms of ARDS include:

- Tachypnea
- Increased work of breathing
- Accessory muscle use
- Hypoxia due to fluid-filled alveoli, preventing effective gas exchange
- Little improvement with oxygenation

Providing 100% oxygen is the mainstay of care. Ventilation may need to be assisted and an advanced airway placed to allow for higher airway pressures to be used. PEEP is also recommended.

Tuberculosis

Older adults are at increased risk of acquiring a tuberculosis (TB) infection due to their decreased immunity and potentially by the communal living in long-term care facilities. Diagnosis is also challenging because showing fewer "classical" signs of infection is a characteristic of the geriatric patient group.

Tuberculosis, caused by infection of the *Mycobacterium tuberculosis* bacterium, typically attacks the lungs but can also infect the spine, brain, or kidneys. Infection can present as latent TB infection or TB disease. Latent TB infection does not make the patient sick or contagious since the patient's immune system keeps the bacteria from growing. TB disease occurs when the immune system is unable to prevent the bacteria from spreading.

The classic signs and symptoms of TB disease include chest pain and persistent cough for 3 or more weeks that produces blood or phlegm. Other signs and symptoms include fatigue, decreased appetite, weight loss, night sweats, fever, and chills.

Treatment for TB can take 4, 6, or 9 months depending on the treatment regimen. Prehospital treatment should focus on increasing oxygenation and preventing the spread of TB. EMS practitioners should wear an N95 respirator when working with patients who have confirmed or suspected TB (**FIGURE 3-10**).

A vaccine for TB is available but is not widely used in the United States. The Bacille Calmette-Guérin (BCG) vaccine should only be considered for at-risk patients and should not be administered without consultation with a TB control program. TB screening should be provided for people with an increased risk for TB disease.

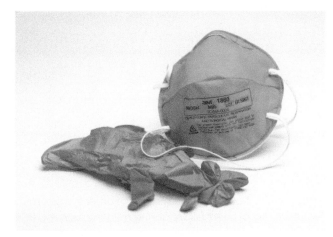

FIGURE 3-10 N95 respirator and gloves.
© Kreative Photography/Shutterstock

Heart Failure/Acute Pulmonary Edema

Heart failure (HF) is a condition of decreased cardiac output due to decreased myocardial contractility, which leads to the inability to maintain metabolic needs. This is often referred to as **pump failure**. Decreased cardiac output at the left ventricle results in inadequate emptying of the ventricle with each contraction. Because less blood is needed to refill the ventricle, blood backs up into the left atrium and the veins and capillaries of the pulmonary system. This results in high intravascular pressures, which force fluid out of the capillaries of the lungs and into the alveolar space. The gas exchange is impaired as alveolar space is filled with fluid. Noncardiac causes of HF in the geriatric population include anemia, renal insufficiency, and hyperthyroidism.

Acute pulmonary edema (APE) is buildup of fluid in the alveoli. HF can cause APE, as can pneumonia, toxins, medications, chest wall trauma, and exertion at high elevations.

The New York Heart Association has classified presentations of HF to assist trending patient conditions (**TABLE 3-4**).

Signs and symptoms of HF can include:

- Dyspnea
- Crackles or rhonchi heard on auscultation
- Jugular vein distension

TABLE 3-4 New York Heart Association Heart Failure Classification Scheme

Class	Clinical Features
I	Patients are generally asymptomatic with exertion.
II	Patients have dyspnea or other symptoms of heart failure during normal exertion.
III	Patients have dyspnea or other symptoms of heart failure during mild exertion.
IV	Patients have symptoms of heart failure with any physical activity.

© Jones & Bartlett Learning

- Hypertension (BP > 160/100 to < 180/120)
- Peripheral edema
- Coughing or shortness of breath when supine
- Increased hepatojugular reflex
- Pulmonary edema without positional dyspnea

Due to changes associated with aging, geriatric patients can tolerate lower blood concentrations of oxygen and higher blood concentrations of carbon dioxide. Therefore, when geriatric patients become symptomatic

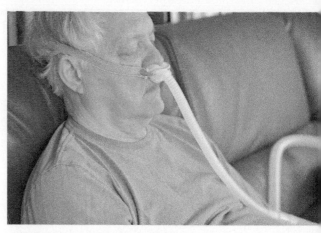

FIGURE 3-11 Position patient sitting upright with CPAP to utilize as much alveolar space as possible.
© Alice Day/Shutterstock

of hypoxia and hypercapnia, they are much more ill than a younger patient.

The treatment goal is to improve the pumping function of the heart by reducing the amount of blood returning to the heart and reducing the pressure, against which the left ventricle must push blood out. This can be done in the prehospital setting with administration of nitroglycerin and CPAP. High-flow oxygen is needed to reverse hypoxia. The patient must be positioned sitting upright to enlist as much alveolar space as possible since the fluid in the spaces will settle to the lower lungs due to gravity (**FIGURE 3-11**).

CASE STUDY

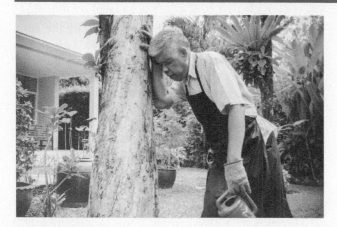

FIGURE 3-12
© chalermphon_tiam/Shutterstock

You and your partner are staffing an emergency response ambulance and are dispatched to the house of a 78-year-old patient complaining of shortness of breath (**FIGURE 3-12**).

QUESTIONS

- What is your differential diagnosis?
  - AMI
  - ACS
  - COPD exacerbation
  - Infection
  - Anemia
  - Cardiomyopathy
  - Pneumonia
  - PE
  - Pleurisy
  - Cardiac arrhythmia
- How does the patient's age affect your assessment approach?
  - Given the patient's age, you should include the GEMS Diamond as part of your overall assessment. You should also keep in mind that older patients experience many age-related changes that can affect the respiratory system, and that they also

have reduced reserve capacity when compared with younger patients. Signs and symptoms can be subtle, and body systems other than respiratory can affect breathing.

The scene appears safe as you don your PPE while approaching the house. You are met at the door by the patient. After opening the door, the patient turns and slowly walks to a nearby chair and sits. It appears that the patient is alone. The home is well-kept, and there are no obvious clues to the patient's medical condition; no medical aids are visible.

The patient is an alert, older male who is breathing faster than normal. As you approach the patient, he tells you that he called EMS after becoming progressively short of breath over the last week.

You perform a primary survey which reveals:

- X–No obvious external bleeding.
- A–Patent airway.
- B–Tachypneic with bilateral exhalatory wheezing and rhonchi on his left side when auscultated.

- C–Strong, irregular radial pulse; skin is cool, dry to touch, and capillary refill is less than 2 seconds.
- D–Alert, oriented to self, place, and time; equal and reactive pupils.
- E–No signs of trauma, edema, or rash.

QUESTIONS

- What is the cardinal presentation and the chief complaint?
  - Cardinal presentation: Tachypnea
  - Chief complaint: Dyspnea/shortness of breath

- Are any interventions required before assessment can continue?
- Does this patient require immediate transport, or can you remain on scene and continue your assessment?
  - The patient appears to be stable, so you continue your assessment on scene.

- What further assessments would you like to perform?
  - Detailed history, vital signs, and physical assessment

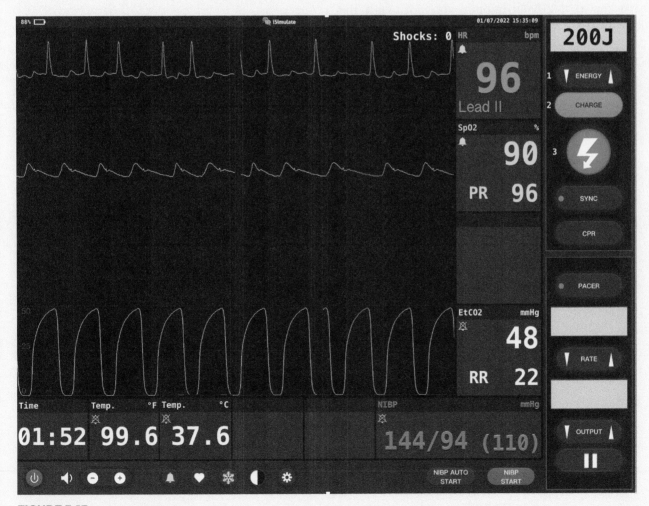

FIGURE 3-13

You further assess the patient by monitoring vital signs, and attaching a cardiac monitor and pulse oximeter to him. The results of these assessments are:

- HR: 96, irregular
- BP: 144/94
- RR: 22
- Temp: 99.6°F (37.5°C) tympanic
- SpO$_2$: 90% on room air
- ECG: is sinus rhythm

Capnometry reads 48 and capnography reveals prolonged expiratory phase and shape consistent with COPD.

A detailed physical assessment reveals no new findings (**FIGURE 3-14**).

The 12-lead ECG shows an irregular rate close to 100 with no acute changes (A-fib).

You elicit the history of the chief complaint and find the onset of symptoms occurred gradually and they have been worsening since. He denies discomfort and is unable to rate the severity of his dyspnea. He says it started a week ago but got worse in the last 45 minutes. Using the OPQRST mnemonic, you document the following information:

- O–Gradual
- P–Aggravated by exertion, nothing relieves it
- Q–N/A
- R–None
- S–Unknown
- T–Started a week ago, but worsened in last 45 minutes

The patient tells you that he feels short of breath, has increased productive cough with a greenish-colored, thick sputum with occasional blood streaks. He admits that he has had limited appetite for the last few days.

The patient does not recall any unusual events leading up to the onset of symptoms a week ago. On this day, he was cleaning the house and doing yard work, but had to stop due to his dyspnea, which set in 45 minutes ago. He has had exertional dyspnea for the last week, but it resolved with rest; however, this current episode would not resolve. The patient lives alone and has no family. He admits to smoking a pack of cigarettes per day for over 25 years.

SAMPLER history is as follows:

- S–Short of breath, increased productive cough with a greenish-colored, thick sputum with occasional blood streaks
- A–None
- M–Salbutamol, fluticasone-umeclidin-vilanter, dextromethorphan-guaifenesin, sotalol, and clopidogrel

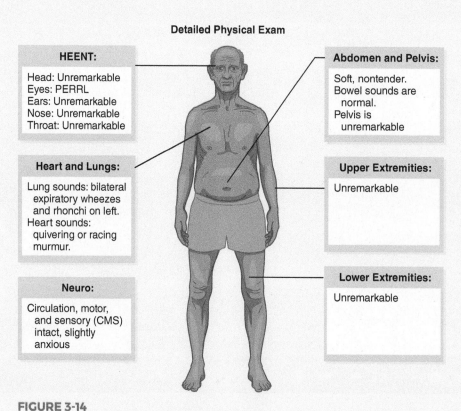

Detailed Physical Exam

HEENT:
Head: Unremarkable
Eyes: PERRL
Ears: Unremarkable
Nose: Unremarkable
Throat: Unremarkable

Heart and Lungs:
Lung sounds: bilateral expiratory wheezes and rhonchi on left.
Heart sounds: quivering or racing murmur.

Neuro:
Circulation, motor, and sensory (CMS) intact, slightly anxious

Abdomen and Pelvis:
Soft, nontender.
Bowel sounds are normal.
Pelvis is unremarkable

Upper Extremities:
Unremarkable

Lower Extremities:
Unremarkable

FIGURE 3-14

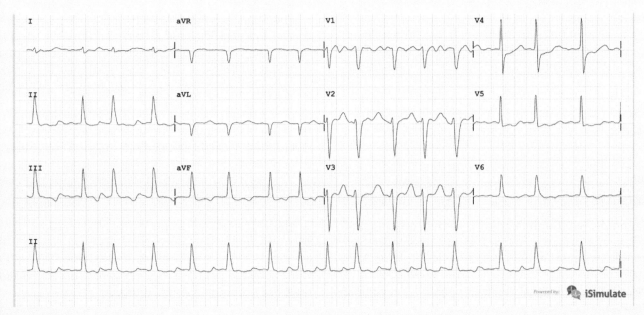

FIGURE 3-15

- P–COPD and atrial fibrillation
- L–Slice of toast an hour ago
- E–No recall of unusual events leading up to the onset of symptoms a week ago. Today, cleaning the house, when dyspnea set in 45 minutes ago
- R–Smoker: pack/day for 25+ years

QUESTIONS

- What are your treatment goals for this patient?
  - Decrease work of breathing, increase oxygenation
  - Monitor patient for any changes or deterioration
  - Deliver appropriate medications to reduce COPD exacerbation

GEMS DIAMOND REVIEW

How was the GEMS Diamond incorporated into the patient assessment?

Geriatric Assessment: The patient is a 78-year-old male with consistent age-related changes.

Environmental Assessment: The home is well-kept with no visible fall hazards noted. The patient appears in good health with no obvious sensory deficits.

Medical Assessment: The patient has a history of COPD and atrial fibrillation. The patient takes multiple medications and confirms he is compliant with taking all of them as directed.

Social Assessment: The patient can accomplish ADLs by himself; he lives alone. He was divorced 25 years ago and has no children.

QUESTIONS

- What does your differential diagnosis include now?
  - ACS
  - Cardiomyopathy
  - COPD exacerbation
  - Dehydration
  - Pneumonia

- What other assessments are likely to be performed in the hospital?
  - Blood tests, chest x-ray, 12-lead ECG

- What treatment should be provided prehospitally?
  - Oxygen administration and IV access established and run at TKVO. Other treatment will vary based on scope of practice and local protocols.

The patient is transported on a stretcher in the Fowler position, to the closest appropriate facility. Oxygen is administered at 4 lpm via nasal cannula and intravenous access is established and run at TKVO. If within scope of practice, bronchodilators, anticholinergics, corticosteroids, and antibiotics should be administered. CPAP and intubation equipment are prepared in case the patient deteriorates during transport.

At the hospital, oxygen and bronchodilator therapy is continued. Blood is drawn and sent to the lab for analysis. A chest x-ray is performed, and a 12-lead ECG repeated.

The final diagnosis for this patient is bacterial pneumonia, dehydration, and COPD exacerbation. He receives fluid therapy to correct the dehydration and antibiotic therapy to treat the pneumonia. He is discharged after a brief stay at the hospital for observation. He is prescribed a course of antibiotics and steroids to help manage his COPD during the antibiotic treatment. He is advised to follow-up with his primary care provider for pneumonia vaccinations and preventive care

CASE STUDY WRAP-UP

Pneumonia is a common disease in the geriatric population due to aging changes to the respiratory and immune systems, more sedentary lifestyle, and lifelong exposure to pollutants. Patients with COPD and atrial fibrillation are at increased risk of developing pneumonias.

Signs of pneumonia can be subtle. Elevated temperatures and productive cough that are common in younger patients are uncommon in older patients. Elevated body temperature in geriatric patients is rare and most likely indicates severe infection.

CHAPTER WRAP-UP

- The geriatric population is at high risk for respiratory disorders and often will have a respiratory component to their medical history.
- Respiratory infections that cause mild illness in younger patients can cause severe to life-threatening illness in those over 65 years of age.

- When signs of respiratory illness become apparent in an older adult patient, the level of illness will be more severe than a younger patient due to the older patient's tolerance for hypoxia and hypercapnia.

REFERENCES

Abbara A, Collin SM, Kon OM, et al. Time to diagnosis of tuberculosis is greater in older patients: a retrospective cohort review. *ERJ Open Res.* 2019 Nov;5(4):00228–2018.

American Lung Association. Asthma-COPD Overlap Syndrome (ACOS). https://www.lung.org/lung-health-diseases/lung-disease-lookup/asthma/diagnosing-treating-asthma/asthma-copd-overlap-syndrome. Updated October 23, 2020. Accessed March 10, 2022.

Arnold FW, Reyes Vega AM, Salunkhe V, et al. Older adults hospitalized for pneumonia in the United States: incidence, epidemiology, and outcomes. *J Am Geriatr Soc.* 2020;68(5):1007–1014. doi:10.1111/jgs.16327

Centers for Disease Control and Prevention. Chest cold (acute bronchitis). https://www.cdc.gov/antibiotic-use/bronchitis.html. Updated July 1, 2021. Accessed March 10, 2022.

Centers for Disease Control and Prevention. Influenza (Flu). https://www.cdc.gov/flu/about/keyfacts.htm. Updated March 14, 2022. Accessed March 10, 2022.

Centers for Disease Control and Prevention. Pneumonia can be prevented—vaccines can help. https://www.cdc.gov/pneumonia/prevention.html. Published October 22, 2018. Accessed May 5, 2021.

Centers for Disease Control and Prevention. Tuberculosis (TB). https://www.cdc.gov/tb/default.htm. Updated March 17, 2022. Accessed March 10, 2022.

Chokroverty S. Sleep disturbances in general medical disorders. *Sleep Disorders Medicine.* Published online 2009:550–580. doi:10.1016/b978-0-7506-7584-0.00033-1

Dhand UK, Goyal M, Sahota P. Sleep-related hypoventilation and hypoxemia due to neuromuscular and chest wall disorders. *Encyclopedia of Sleep.* Published online 2013:325–331. doi:10.1016/b978-0-12-378610-4.00329-6

Dijk FN, de Jongste JC, Postma DS, Koppelman GH. Genetics of onset of asthma. *Curr Opin Allergy Clin Immunol.* 2013 Apr;13(2):193–202. doi:10.1097/ACI.0b013e32835eb707

Elsevier. Deconditioning. Elsevier Health. https://elsevier.health/en-US/preview/deconditioning. Updated May 14, 2020. Accessed March 22, 2022.

Flannery B, Chung JR, Monto AS, et al. Influenza vaccine effectiveness in the United States during the 2016–2017 season. *Clin Infect Dis.* 2019 May;68(11):1798–1806.

Jackson ML, Neuzil KM, Thompson WW, et al. The burden of community-acquired pneumonia in seniors: results of a population-based study. *Clin Infect Dis*. 2004;39(11):1642–1650. doi:10.1086/425615

National Association of Emergency Medical Technicians (NAEMT). *AMLS: Advanced Medical Life Support: An Assessment-Based Approach*. 3rd ed. Burlington, MA: Jones & Bartlett Learning; 2021.

National Heart, Lung, and Blood Institute. COPD. https://www.nhlbi.nih.gov/health-topics/copd. Published 2018. Accessed May 8, 2021.

National Heart, Lung, and Blood institute. Pneumonia. https://www.nhlbi.nih.gov/health-topics/pneumonia. Published 2018. Accessed May 5, 2021.

Nicholson KG. Clinical features of influenza. *Semin Respir Infect*. 1992 Mar;7(1):26–37.

Sharma G, Goodwin J. Effect of aging on respiratory system physiology and immunology. *Clin Interv Aging*. 2006;1(3):253–260. doi:10.2147/ciia.2006.1.3.253

Solomon DA, Sherman AC, Kanjilal S. Influenza in the COVID-19 era. *JAMA*. 2020;324(13):1342–1343. doi:10.1001/jama.2020.14661

Tzortzaki EG, Proklou A, Siafakas NM. Asthma in the elderly: can we distinguish it from COPD? *J Allergy*. 2011;2011:1–7. doi:10.1155/2011/843543

World Health Organization (WHO). The top 10 causes of death. https://www.who.int/news-room/fact-sheets/detail/the-top-10-causes-of-death. Published December 9, 2020. Accessed May 2, 2021.

CHAPTER 4

Cardiovascular Emergencies

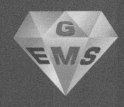

LESSON OBJECTIVES

- Review the anatomy and physiology of the heart.
- Discuss the epidemiology, pathophysiology, assessment, and treatment of older patients with cardiovascular emergencies.
- Identify the signs and symptoms and medications that could impact the aging population experiencing a cardiovascular emergency.

Introduction

Cardiovascular disease is the most common medical condition in the adult population over 65 years. As the American population ages, heart disease will become the most common medical complaint EMS is called to treat. In the 60 to 79-year-old age group in America, 77.2% of men and 78.2% of women have heart disease. For adults 80 years of age and older, those numbers jump to 89.3% and 92.8%, respectively.

The World's #1 Killer

Cardiovascular disease is the leading cause of death in people older than 65 years (in addition to being the leading cause of death overall in both the United States and worldwide).

Cardiovascular Disease in the Older Adult

Aging is associated with predictable anatomic and physiologic changes to the cardiovascular system. Because of these changes, cardiovascular disease will not manifest the same clinical features in older patients as in younger patients. Additionally, prescribed medications and comorbidities also complicate the assessment of this type of patient.

Chronic high blood pressure causes hypertensive heart disease as people get older. The risk of heart failure due to hypertensive heart disease for those over 65 years is doubled for men and tripled for women. Hypertensive heart disease puts the elderly patient at risk for heart failure (HF), acute coronary syndrome, and sudden cardiac death.

The Silent Killer

Chronic untreated high blood pressure is asymptomatic but causes cardiac changes that greatly increase the risk of serious heart disease with age.

Cardiac Anatomy and Physiology

The heart is primarily composed of a unique type of muscle tissue that can initiate a contraction without an external stimulus. Contraction of the heart is coordinated to pump more blood efficiently using a system of heart muscle tissue with a faster conductivity than normal heart muscle tissue. Each heartbeat is initiated by

Heart Anatomy

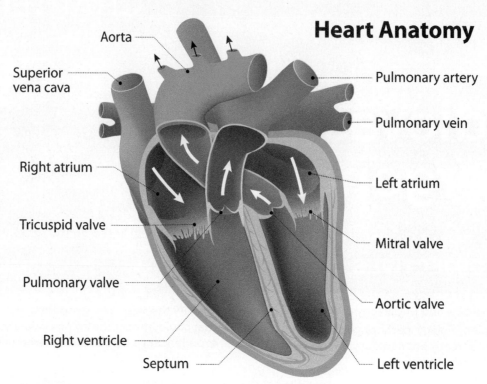

FIGURE 4-1 Anatomy of the human heart and direction of blood flow.
© Designua/Shutterstock

a group of muscle cells in the right atria that self-excite much faster than other cells of the heart. This group of cardiac muscle cells, or pacemaker cells, is called the sinoatrial (SA) node (**FIGURE 4-1**).

Hearts Are Lefties

The left ventricle makes up most of the heart's mass. The right ventricle has much thinner walls than the left because it pumps blood to the lower-pressure pulmonary circuit.

The right coronary artery (RCA) supplies the right side of the heart and the inferior left ventricular wall in most people. The left coronary artery (LCA) feeds most of the left side of the heart. The LCA branches into the left anterior descending (LAD) and the left circumflex arteries (LCX). The LAD feeds most of the interventricular septum and both anterior ventricles. It is responsible for feeding most of the left ventricular muscle

The Widow Maker

Blockage of the LAD is associated with high rates of cardiac arrest.

mass. The LCX feeds the left atrium and posterior left ventricle regions.

Injured, dying, and dead heart tissue will cause changes to the pacemaker impulse conduction patterns. Because the conduction system and coronary circulation are similar from person to person, changes in the impulse conduction can identify which coronary artery is obstructed. A 12-lead ECG provides enough electrical views of the heart to do this (**TABLE 4-1**).

These 12 leads can be augmented by the placement of additional leads to view the posterior and right side of the heart, as shown in **TABLE 4-2**.

Common Pathologies
Valvular Heart Disease
Aortic Valve

Degenerative changes to this valve are common in the geriatric patient. The aortic valve is the one-way valve that allows blood to exit the left ventricle and enter the aorta during ventricular contraction. It is composed of three thin, flexible flaps or leaflets. Age-related changes involve the thickening, calcification, and fusion of the leaflets. **Aortic stenosis** occurs when the valve becomes unable to completely open during ventricular contraction, inhibiting blood flow out of the chamber. **Aortic regurgitation** occurs when the valve does not

TABLE 4-1 12-Lead ECG Leads by Region to Identify Coronary Artery Obstruction

Region	Coronary Artery	ECG Lead
SA node	RCA	I, II
AV node	RCA (75%); LAD (25%)	II
Right atria, right ventricle, inferior left ventricle	RCA	II, III, aVF
Septum, anterior left ventricle	LAD	V1, V2, V3, V4
Left atrium, posterior left ventricle	LCX; RCA	I, aVL, V5, V6
No associated region		aVR

Copyright © 2024 National Association of Emergency Medical Technicians (NAEMT).

TABLE 4-2 Additional Leads to View the Posterior and Right Side of the Heart

Region	Coronary Artery	ECG Lead
Posterior left ventricle	LCX, RCA	V7, V8, V9
Right ventricle	RCA	V4R, V5R, V6R

Copyright © 2024 National Association of Emergency Medical Technicians (NAEMT).

Age-Related Cardiovascular Changes

Most age-related cardiovascular change occurs due to atherosclerosis in the geriatric population (**TABLE 4-3**). Refer to Chapter 1: Changes with Age for more detailed discussion of these changes.

Common Arrythmias

The most common arrythmias in older adults are atrial fibrillation, bradyarrhythmia, conduction system disorders (including bundle branch block, heart block, and long QT syndrome), supraventricular arrythmias, and ventricular arrythmias.

TABLE 4-3 Age-Related Cardiovascular Changes and Their Resulting Pathologies

Age-Related Changes	Results
Atherosclerosis	Hypertension
	Heart failure
SA node deterioration	Arrythmias
Conduction system degradation	
Aortic stenosis	Heart failure
	Cerebrovascular accident (CVA)
	Arrythmias
	Cardiac infection
Valve calcification	Arrythmias
	Myocardial infarction
	CVA
Decreased sensitivity of baroreceptors	Orthostatic hypotension

Copyright © 2024 National Association of Emergency Medical Technicians (NAEMT).

completely close when the ventricle relaxes. This allows the blood to re-enter the ventricle after contraction from both the aorta and the left atrium instead of solely the left atrium.

Both conditions reduce ventricular emptying and cardiac output. This can cause symptoms such as chest pain, tachycardia, dyspnea, dizziness, syncope, and pedal edema.

Mitral Valve

The mitral valve allows the one-way flow of blood out of the left atrium into the left ventricle. This valve is structurally very different to the aortic valve and contains only two leaflets. Like the aortic valve, the mitral valve can also suffer the degenerative changes but more often damage occurs at younger ages due to infection, autoimmune disorder, or other disease processes. As with the aortic valve, **mitral stenosis** (**FIGURE 4-2**) involves reduced valve opening and **mitral regurgitation** involves incomplete valve closure.

Both mitral valve conditions reduce pumping function of the left ventricle and therefore decrease cardiac output. Some symptoms of mitral stenosis are like

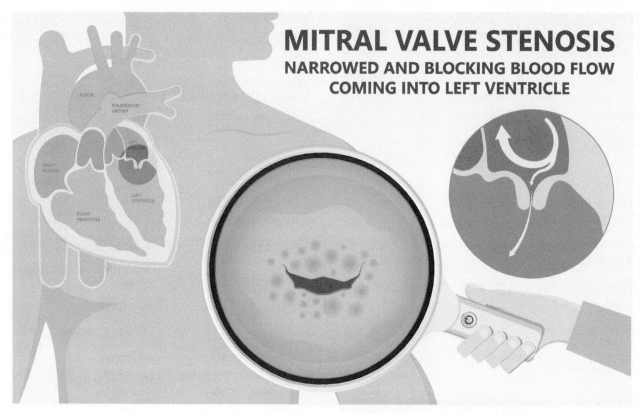

MITRAL VALVE STENOSIS
NARROWED AND BLOCKING BLOOD FLOW COMING INTO LEFT VENTRICLE

FIGURE 4-2 Narrowed blood flow into the left ventricle, indicative of mitral valve stenosis.
© Pepermpron/Shutterstock

those of aortic valve dysfunction and include chest pain, tachycardia, dizziness, pedal edema, and syncope (**FIGURE 4-3**). Other clinical features may include exertional dyspnea, dyspnea when supine, fatigue, and coughing up blood from the respiratory tract, either small amounts in sputum or large amounts with a forceful cough. Symptoms of mitral regurgitation include irregular heartbeat, difficulty breathing especially when lying flat, fatigue, and pedal edema.

Prehospital Management of Valvular Disease

Symptoms of valvular disease are so similar to other cardiac complaints that the EMS practitioner may not be aware of the true nature of the complaint until hospital investigation and diagnosis are completed. Therefore, the care will be the same as for other more common cardiac complaints such as acute coronary syndromes or acute heart failure.

As with the other cardiac conditions, care is primarily aimed at maintaining airway, breathing, and circulation. Oxygen should be provided to reverse hypoxia or dyspnea, pain relief provided as needed, volume resuscitation initiated to improve cardiac output, and any arrythmias managed. Patients in respiratory distress may also benefit from CPAP (**FIGURE 4-4**).

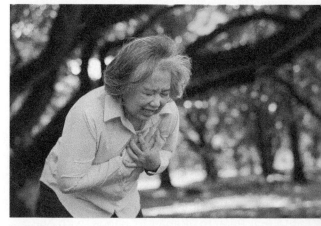

FIGURE 4-3 Mitral valve stenosis symptoms can include chest pain, tachycardia, dizziness, pedal edema, and syncope.
© PattyPhoto/Shutterstock

Treat the Failure

In the prehospital setting, you can determine a patient is in heart failure but not diagnose the cause. Treating the signs and symptoms of heart failure is appropriate EMS care for a patient with valvular disease.

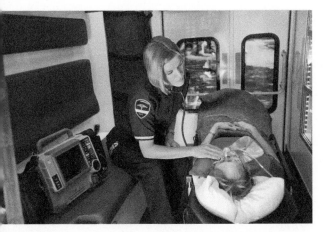

FIGURE 4-4 Prehospital management of valvular disease may involve oxygenation to reverse hypoxia or dyspnea.
© Tyler Olson/Shutterstock

Heart Failure

The heart can structurally and functionally be divided into the left and the right, with the left side pumping blood from the lungs to the body, and the right side pumping blood from the body to the lungs. When the heart becomes damaged and begins to fail, it can be right-sided failure, left-sided failure, or both. HF can have a variable presentation depending on the degree of failure and which side of the heart is affected (**FIGURE 4-5**).

Heart failure is discussed in Chapter 3 in the Heart Failure/Acute Pulmonary Edema section; **TABLE 4-4** compares the effects and features of right- and left-sided heart failure.

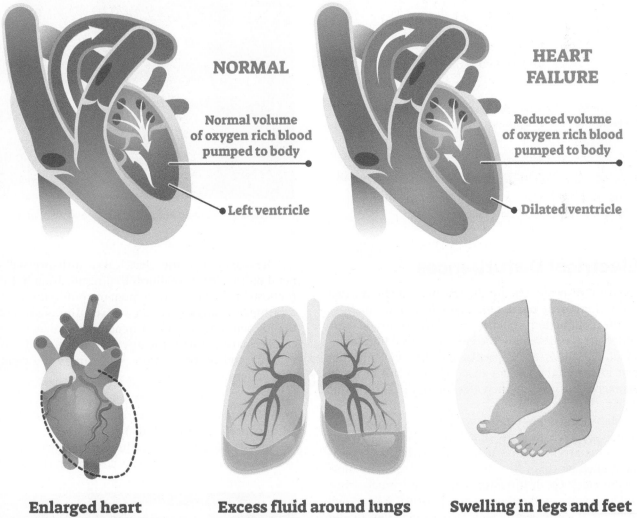

Enlarged heart Chest congestion

Excess fluid around lungs Shortness of breath

Swelling in legs and feet Edema

FIGURE 4-5 Normal heart versus heart failure. Note fluid retention in both the lungs and extremities.
© VectorMine/Shutterstock

TABLE 4-4 Right- versus Left-Sided Heart Failure: Effects and Clinical Features

Type of Failure	Effect	Clinical Features
Right-sided	Impaired pumping of the right ventricle Buildup of fluid into the peripheral body tissues	Pedal or sacral edema Ascites Dyspnea Chest pain Palpitations
Left-sided	Impaired pumping of the left ventricle Buildup of fluid into the alveoli, leading to pulmonary edema	Persistent coughing Nocturnal dyspnea Exertional dyspnea Weight gain Arrythmias

Copyright © 2024 National Association of Emergency Medical Technicians (NAEMT).

Failure Leads to Failure

The most common cause of right-sided heart failure is left-sided heart failure.

Electrical Disturbances

Electrical disturbances are disturbances in the normal heart rhythm or heart rate, caused by abnormalities in the conduction system. The most common sustained arrythmia among the elderly is atrial fibrillation (A-fib). A-fib is an unpredictable, irregular rhythm that increases the risk for blood clots. If not properly managed, this rhythm increases the risk of thrombotic stroke.

Many arrythmias can be asymptomatic or have mild symptoms such as sinus bradycardia, sinus tachycardia, sinus arrythmia, normal sinus rhythm with bundle branch block, or first-degree heart block. The most severe electrical disturbances can cause cardiac arrest suddenly and without warning (**FIGURE 4-6**). Such rhythms include ventricular tachycardia, ventricular fibrillation, and asystole. Recognizing an unresponsive patient with absent breathing and pulse is critical to begin effective care.

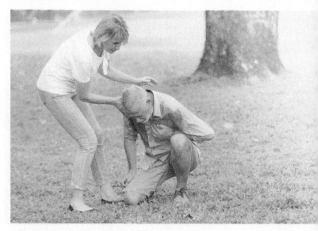

FIGURE 4-6 Severe electrical disturbances can cause cardiac arrest suddenly and without warning.
© P.KASIPAT/Shutterstock

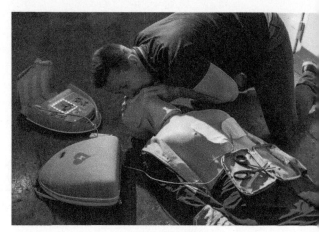

FIGURE 4-7 Use of an automatic external defibrillator.
© Egor_Kulinich/Shutterstock

Management of the electrical disturbance will depend on the degree of illness that results from it. In the prehospital setting, management of nonlife-threatening arrythmias is supportive care with continuous monitoring for deterioration. Life-threatening cardiac rhythms can be managed with therapy intended to end the arrythmia and restore a more stable perfusing conduction pattern:

- CPR
- AED/cardiac monitor as early as possible (**FIGURE 4-7**)
- Advanced airway and medications
- Transport to advanced/definitive cardiovascular care
- Early return of spontaneous circulation (ROSC) care

Critical Thinking Question

What is the fastest way to stop a lethal, non-perfusing cardiac rhythm?

Hypertensive Emergencies

A **hypertensive emergency** is differentiated from hypertension by the presence of signs or symptoms of organ damage due to the elevated blood pressure. Patients with chronic hypertension may not exhibit any signs or symptoms until the systolic pressure is significantly elevated.

There are two types of hypertension: primary and secondary. Primary hypertension develops over time and has no one identifiable cause, while secondary hypertension is due to another condition and can occur without warning.

Secondary hypertension usually appears with higher blood pressure than primary hypertension. Many conditions and medications can lead to secondary hypertension, including obstructive sleep apnea, adrenal gland tumors, kidney disease, thyroid conditions, congenital blood vessel defects, a host of medications (both OTC and prescription), and illicit drug use.

Clinical features can include chest pain, headache, nausea, vomiting, anxiety, bounding and rapid heart rate, tinnitus, difficulty breathing, spontaneous nosebleed, altered mental status, and seizure. Prehospital management of this type of patient is supportive (**FIGURE 4-8**). Aggressive attempts to lower blood pressure are typically unnecessary in asymptomatic patients and could lead to hypotension. Patients should be transported with the head elevated.

Syncope

Many different mechanisms can be responsible for syncope in the geriatric population. For instance, syncope can be due to a neurologic problem such as a transient ischemic attack, a cardiac problem such as arrythmia, orthostatic hypotension, dehydration, or medication toxicity.

Not "Just a Fainting Spell"

Always assume an older person's syncopal episode suggests a life-threatening condition until proven otherwise.

Assessment of a geriatric patient who has experienced a syncopal episode is more complex than the typical medical approach. A thorough description of the event, including presyncopal complaints, duration of episode, patient behavior during the episode, and patient's recovery from the event, can be helpful. The patient should be assessed for any persisting complaints such as altered mentation, lightheadedness, dizziness, vision changes, and balance difficulty. If the syncopal episode involved a fall or other trauma (**FIGURE 4-9**), thoroughly assess the patient for injury no matter how minor the mechanism of injury appears to be. Prehospital management of this type of patient will be guided by the assessment findings.

Coronary Artery Disease

Coronary artery disease (CAD) is the most common type of heart disease and the leading cause of death in the United States. (If a patient tells you that they have "heart disease," they are very likely referring to CAD.) CAD results in impaired coronary blood flow due to the build-up of cholesterol and other fatty substances on the inside walls of blood vessels feeding the heart (**FIGURE 4-10**). This collection of material damages the blood vessel walls, inhibiting the ability to dilate and

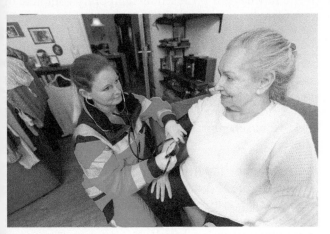

FIGURE 4-8 Continue to monitor the patient's blood pressure, as patients with chronic hypertension may not exhibit any signs or symptoms until the systolic pressure is significantly elevated.
© Nehris/Shutterstock

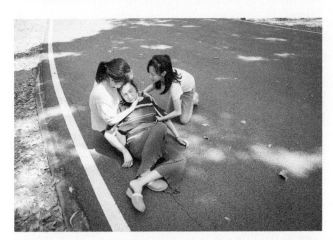

FIGURE 4-9 Patients suffering a syncopal episode may fall due to lightheadedness, dizziness, and balance difficulties. Be sure to assess the patient for injury.
© CGN089/Shutterstock

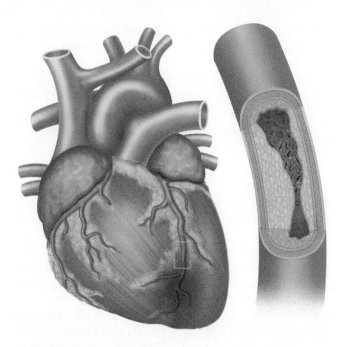

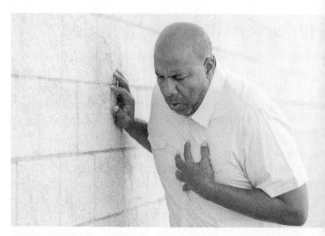

FIGURE 4-11 In unstable angina, pain is more severe than in angina pectoris.
© pixelheadphoto digitalskillet/Shutterstock

FIGURE 4-10 Build-up of cholesterol and other fatty substances along the walls of blood vessels eventually leads to the body's flow needs not being met.
© ilusmedical/Shutterstock

increase blood flow and oxygen delivery when needed. Major risk factors include smoking, hypertension, high cholesterol, and diabetes.

Atherosclerosis versus Arteriosclerosis

Atherosclerosis is the accumulation of fats, cholesterol, and other substances on and in the inner lining of arterial walls throughout the body. Atherosclerosis is a type of **arteriosclerosis**, which involves the thickening and stiffening of arterial walls.

Acute Coronary Syndrome

Acute coronary syndrome (ACS) describes the group of symptoms related to acute myocardial ischemia. ACS includes three progressive conditions: angina pectoris, unstable angina, and acute myocardial infarction. Cardiac observation is needed in all three conditions, as ACS requires greater coronary oxygen demand than the patient could provide.

Angina Pectoris

Commonly referred to simply as angina, angina pectoris involves brief episodes of chest pain. Symptoms occur when increased of demand for oxygen by cardiac muscle is not met. This may be due to narrowing of the artery lumen or inability of the coronary arteries to

dilate. The discomfort is typically described as a crushing, squeezing, or pressure sensation that may radiate to the arms, jaw, midback, or epigastrium. The pain is predictably induced by exertion and resolves with rest after a brief period of 3 to 8 minutes. Pain rarely lasts longer than 15 minutes. Other symptoms can include nausea, sweating, and shortness of breath. Patients typically manage this complaint with rest and prescribed nitroglycerin administration.

Unstable Angina

Unstable angina represents a progressive deterioration of angina in which the predictability of symptom onset is no longer reliable. Unstable angina can occur when the patient is at rest and is more persistent, lasting longer than 15 minutes (**FIGURE 4-11**). A patient may describe the pain as increasing in duration and intensity over a few days. It is caused by temporary complete or near complete blockage of a coronary artery.

A rare variant of angina that presents much like unstable angina is **Prinzmetal angina**. This condition involves coronary artery spasm and can be caused by cold weather exposure, stress, medicines, smoking, and cocaine use. It usually occurs while at rest or during the night and usually the pain is severe. Nitroglycerin is effective in relaxing the spasm and resolving the chest pain.

Acute Myocardial Infarction

Acute myocardial infarction (AMI) is caused by a clot. If a coronary artery becomes completely obstructed, the cardiac cells in the heart muscle will die, releasing intracellular materials into the bloodstream. These proteins, called troponins, are cardiac biomarkers that can be identified in a blood sample and aid in the diagnosis of AMI. Death of heart muscle will also disrupt the normal electrical pattern 15 minutes after onset to allow for a rapid and noninvasive determination of AMI by 12-lead ECG. Based on the blood analysis and ECG evaluation, AMI can be categorized as non–ST-elevation MI (NSTE-ACS) and **ST-elevation MI (STEMI)**.

Hard to Tell

It is difficult to differentiate between unstable angina and acute myocardial infarction without 12-lead ECG and blood analysis.

In addition to the clinical features of angina, patients with NSTE-ACS have ST segment depression or prominent T wave inversion on their ECG and positive cardiac necrosis biomarkers in their blood sample.

12-Lead ECG Is Not a Catchall

Because 12-lead ECG changes are not specific to myocardial infarction, analysis of blood samples are needed to make the correct diagnosis for the NSTE-ACS patient.

STEMI symptoms are highly variable and can range from severe discomfort to a general and mild feeling of being unwell. STEMI is diagnosed based on suspicious symptoms and risk factors accompanied by persistent ST elevation on the ECG and positive cardiac necrosis biomarkers in the blood sample.

The specific region of cardiac infarction can be determined by the electrical changes and corresponding pattern changes on the 12-lead ECG (**FIGURE 4-12**, **TABLE 4-5**).

Recall that the RCA feeds the SA node, right ventricle, and inferior wall of the left ventricle in most people. An ECG indicating an inferior wall AMI could also indicate a right ventricular AMI. Since a patient with right ventricular AMI is susceptible to hypotension causing decreased cardiac perfusion, assess the right-side leads to determine if right ventricular AMI is present.

Critical Thinking Question

Why is an inferior wall AMI often associated with bradyarrhythmias, including heart blocks?

ST Elevated Myocardial Infarction (STEMI)

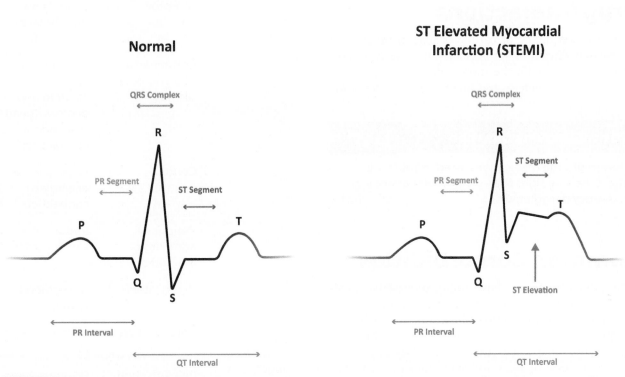

FIGURE 4-12 STEMI can be seen on a 12-lead ECG—notice the ST elevation on the right side of the image compared to the normal ST segment on the left.

TABLE 4-5 Region of Cardiac Infarction by Corresponding 12-Lead ECG Patterns

Region of MI	ECG Leads Affected
Lateral	ST elevation: I, aVL, V5, V6 ST depression: II, III, aVF
Inferior	ST elevation: II, III, aVF ST depression: I, aVL
Septal	ST elevation: V1, V2 ST depression: V7, V8, V9
Anterior	ST elevation: V3. V4
Anteroseptal	ST elevation V1, V2, V3, V4
Posterior	ST elevation: V7, V8, V9 ST depression: V1, V2
Right ventricular	ST elevation: V4R, V5R, V6R, II, III, aVF ST depression: V1, aVL

Copyright © 2024 National Association of Emergency Medical Technicians (NAEMT).

Drug Interactions

Given the frequency of cardiovascular disorders and the use of medications in the elderly, it is useful to have some familiarity with the more common medications prescribed to the elderly and their effects (**TABLE 4-6**).

Critical Thinking Question

How might the medications listed in Table 4-6 affect the vital signs of an older adult patient who is severely dehydrated?

Common Comorbidities

Older adults frequently have noncardiovascular medical comorbidities. Patient adherence to therapeutic guidelines for ACS is also subpar in these patients. The presence of noncardiovascular comorbidities can impact your assessment findings as they may alter the presentation of signs and symptoms of cardiovascular emergencies. Comorbidities also influence the short-term prognosis in ACS patients. Noncardiovascular comorbidities are associated with higher in-hospital mortality.

TABLE 4-6 Cardiac Medications Classification and Effects

Use of Medication	Classification of Medication	Effects of Medication
Blood pressure control	Diuretics	Decrease the amount of fluid in the vascular space and excess fluid secreted
	Beta blockers	Decrease heart rate and force of cardiac contraction
	ACE inhibitors	Inhibit blood vessel constriction
	Angiotensin II receptor blockers	Causes vasodilation by blocking angiotensin II
	Calcium channel blockers	Reduce heart rate and contraction force
	Alpha-2 receptor agonists	Decrease central and peripheral sympathetic flow
	Combined alpha and beta blockers	Inhibit blood vessel constriction and decrease heart rate and force of contraction
	Central agonists	Reduce force of cardiac contraction
	Peripheral adrenergic inhibitors	Reduce vasoconstriction
	Vasodilators	Dilate blood vessels
Heart rate regulation	Beta blockers	Decrease heart rate
	Calcium channel blockers	Decrease heart rate

Copyright © 2024 National Association of Emergency Medical Technicians (NAEMT).

Comorbidities vary by patient; however, there are clusters of comorbidities that are more prevalent than others. See **BOX 4-1** for a list of noncardiovascular comorbidities.

TABLES 4-7, 4-8, and **4-9** provide a contrast and comparison of cardiac conditions covered in this lesson.

BOX 4-1 Common Cormorbidities

- Chronic kidney diseases
- Respiratory/pulmonary diseases
  - COPD
  - Asthma
- Musculoskeletal conditions
  - Osteoporosis and osteoarthritis
  - Hernia
  - Spondylarthritis
  - Scoliosis
- Low vision
  - Retinopathy
  - Macular degeneration
  - Glaucoma
  - Cataract
  - Blindness
- Metabolic
  - Obesity
- Endocrine disorders
  - Diabetes
- Cancer
- Mental health
  - Depression
  - Dementia

TABLE 4-7 Valvular Heart Disease

Condition	Aortic stenosis and aortic regurgitation	Mitral stenosis	Mitral regurgitation	Treatment
Symptoms	Chest pain	Chest pain	Chest pain	■ Focus on: – Circulation – Airway – Breathing ■ Provide: – Pain management – Volume resuscitation to improve cardiac output – Oxygenation ■ Manage dysrhythmia according to local protocols ■ Respiratory distress → CPAP
	Rapid heart rate	Rapid heart rate	Rapid heart rate	
	Difficulty breathing	Difficulty breathing w/ exertion or when lying flat	Difficulty breathing w/exertion or lying flat	
	Dizziness	Dizziness	Dizziness	
		Fatigue	Fatigue	
	Syncope	Syncope	Syncope	
		Hemoptysis	Hemoptysis	
	Pedal edema	Pedal edema	Pedal edema	

TABLE 4-8 Coronary Artery Disease and Electrical Disturbances

Condition	Coronary artery disease (atherosclerosis)	Atrial fibrillation and cardiac arrest	Hypertensive emergencies	Syncope
Symptoms	Chest pain	Chest pain	Chest pain	
	Headache		Headache	
		Shortness of breath		Lightheadedness
	Nausea		Nausea	
	Bounding and rapid heart rate	Rapid heart rate	Bounding and rapid heart rate	
	Vomiting		Vomiting	
		Fatigue		Blacking out
	Anxiety		Anxiety	
	Tinnitus		Tinnitus	
		Persistent cough		Dizziness
		Wheezing		Vision changes
		Pedal edema		Balance problems
	Difficulty breathing	Difficulty breathing	Difficulty breathing	
	Nosebleed		Nosebleed	
	AMS		AMS	AMS
	Seizure		Seizure	
Treatment	■ CPR ■ AED/cardiac monitor as early as possible ■ Advanced airway and medications ■ Transport to advanced/definitive cardiovascular care ■ Early return of spontaneous circulation (ROSC) care	■ CPR ■ AED/cardiac monitor as early as possible ■ Advanced airway and medications ■ Transport to advanced/definitive cardiovascular care ■ Early return of spontaneous circulation (ROSC) care	■ Maintain level of comfort with head elevated ■ **Caution:** aggressive attempts to ↓ blood pressure are unnecessary in asymptomatic patients → hypotension	■ **Syncope = life threatening** ■ Physical exam + focused history ■ Management focused on exam findings

TABLE 4-9 Acute Coronary Syndrome

Acute Coronary Syndrome			
Condition	*Angina Pectoris*	*Unstable Angina*	*Acute Myocardial Infarction*
Symptoms	Brief chest discomfort	Pain > 15 minutes More severe Increased intensity over days Not relieved with rest	Hypotension
	Crushing, squeezing, or pressure to substernal region	Crushing, squeezing, or pressure to substernal region	Elevated jugular venous pressure
	Radiating pain	Radiating pain	Clear and equal lung fields bilaterally
	Nausea	Nausea	
	Sweating	Sweating	
	Shortness of breath	Shortness of breath	
Treatment	▪ Cardiac observation ▪ Rest, oxygen, and/or nitroglycerin	▪ Cardiac observation	▪ Cardiac observation ▪ **Caution!** Administering opiates or nitrates could exacerbate the disorder ▪ **Look!** Ischemia could interfere with normal electrical patterns → significant heart block

Copyright © 2024 National Association of Emergency Medical Technicians (NAEMT).

CASE STUDY

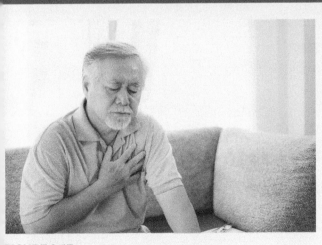

FIGURE 4-13

It is 2100 on a cool spring evening. You and your partner are staffing an emergency response ambulance and are dispatched to the home of a 65-year-old male patient complaining of chest pain.

QUESTIONS

- What is your differential diagnosis?
  - AMI
  - ACS
  - Gastritis
  - Ulcer
  - Thoracic aortic dissection
  - Heart failure
  - GERD
  - Cardiomyopathy
  - Pleurisy
  - Trauma (pneumothorax)

- How does the patient's age affect your assessment approach?
  - You decide to include the GEMS Diamond as part of your overall assessment.

The scene appears safe as you don your PPE while approaching the house. You are met at the door by the patient's wife. She appears anxious and tells you that her husband was watching TV in his recliner after dinner when the chest pain started.

She leads you to the patient—a heavy-set man, alert and breathing normally. His skin appears pale. As you approach the patient, he smiles and tells you that he asked her to call EMS because the pain has persisted and worsened over the last few hours. He says he took baby aspirin and two doses of his nitroglycerin spray and had no relief.

QUESTION

- Do you have any concerns based on your findings so far?
  - Chest pain could be a sign of an acute MI.
  - Chest pain is a common symptom of a heart attack in the geriatric population.

You perform the primary survey, which reveals the following:

- X–No bleeding
- A–Patent airway
- B–Breathing normally with no adventitious sounds when auscultated
- C–Palpable radial pulse, which is regular; skin is cool and dry to touch
- D–Alert; oriented to self, place, and time; and has equal and reactive pupils
- E–Quick assessment reveals no signs of trauma, edema, or rash

He complains of no other symptoms and shares a history of coronary artery disease, hypertension, and hyperlipidemia. He is compliant with his prescriptions of nitroglycerin, aspirin, atenolol, and atorvastatin. He last ate a cheese sandwich and soup about 3 hours ago.

The patient does not recall any unusual events leading up to the sudden onset of pain, which started about 3 hours ago and has been worsening since. His medications have provided no relief. Usually, his pain

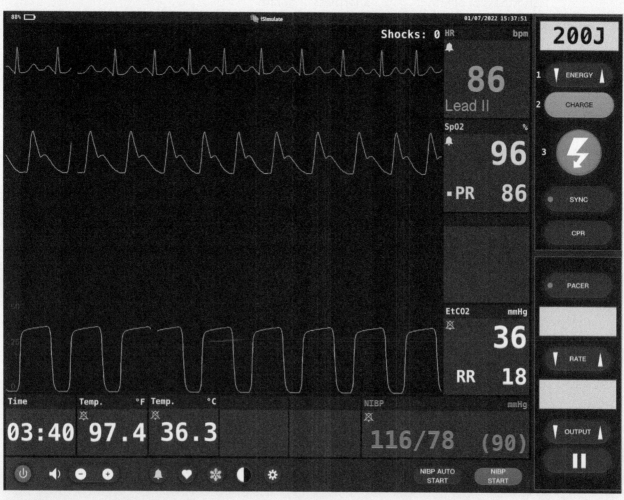

FIGURE 4-14

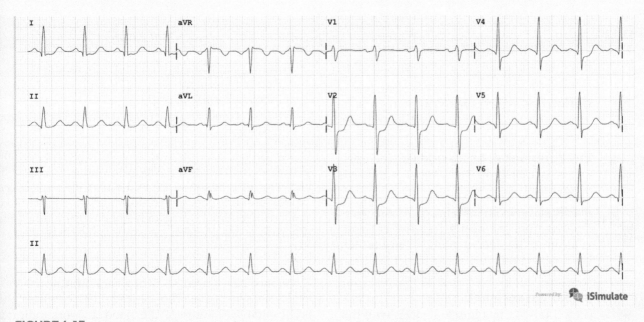

FIGURE 4-15

starts with exertion and is resolved after 2 doses of nitroglycerin. He is not sure if anything makes the pain
worse as he has remained in his chair. He describes the
pain as a substernal 8/10 non-radiating pressure and
different in nature than his typical angina pain. The
patient lives fully independently with his wife and has
no other family.

A brief head-to-toe examination is unremarkable.

QUESTIONS

- What is the cardinal presentation and the chief
  complaint?
  - Cardinal presentation: Chest pain
  - Chief complaint: Chest pain
  - For some patients, the cardinal presentation and
    chief complaint might be the same.
- Are there any life threats identified in this case?
  - This patient is exhibiting signs of chest pain,
    potentially indicating a life threat but additional
    examination is needed.
- Does this patient require immediate transport, or can
  you remain on scene and continue your assessment?
  - The patient is presently stable, so you can continue
    your assessment on scene.
- What further assessments would you like to
  perform?
  - Detailed history, vital signs, physical assessment

You use the OPQRST mnemonic to assess the characteristics of the patient's symptoms.

- O–3 hours ago after eating dinner in the evening

- P–Sitting in recliner watching TV
- Q–Constant, increasing in intensity, different in
  nature from his typical angina pain
- R–Nonradiating, substernal
- S–The patient rates the pain as 8/10
- T–Increasing pain despite medication to treat pain
  over the past few hours

You elicit the history of the cardinal presentation as
best you can using the SAMPLER mnemonic.

- S–Alert, worsening chest pain that is not relieved
  with medication and rest
- A–No known drug allergies
- M–Nitroglycerin, aspirin, atenolol, and atorvastatin
- P–Obesity, coronary artery disease, hypertension,
  and hyperlipidemia
- L–A cheese sandwich and soup about 3 hours ago
- E–Sitting in recliner watching TV after eating dinner
- R–Age, cardiac conditions

You further assess the patient by measuring blood
pressure and attaching a cardiac monitor and oximeter.
The results of these assessments:

- HR: 86, irregular
- BP: 116/78
- RR: 18
- Temp: 97.4°F (36.3°C) tympanic
- SpO$_2$: 96% on room air
- ECG: sinus rhythm

A 12-lead ECG reveals small pathologic Q waves in
leads III and aVF along with ST depression in leads V5
and V6, plus T wave inversion in leads II, III, and aVF.

GEMS DIAMOND REVIEW

How was the GEMS Diamond information applied in this case?

Geriatric Assessment: The patient is a 65-year-old male with expected age-related changes.

Environmental Assessment: The residence is well-kept. The patient is dressed appropriately.

Medical Assessment: In addition to your findings from the detailed assessment and vital signs, the patient advises you that he has been taking his medications as prescribed, but they did not work this time.

Social Assessment: The patient can accomplish ADLs by himself; he lives with his wife. They take care of themselves and have no family nearby.

QUESTIONS

- What other assessments are likely to be performed in the hospital?
  - An additional 12-lead ECG (to check for changes from the one you performed), as well as blood work to check for elevated cardiac enzymes.
- What is your goal for prehospital treatment?
  - Pain management
  - Increase cardiac perfusion
  - Rapid transport to a facility with cardiac catheterization capabilities

The patient is transported on a stretcher in a position of comfort to the closest facility with cardiac care capabilities. Aspirin is administered to the total dose prescribed by local protocol. Nitroglycerin 0.4 mg SL is administered along with fentanyl 1 mcg/kg IVP and ondansetron 4 mg IVP. The patient is monitored continuously during transport and the patient reports that his pain is reduced to 2/10 on arrival at the emergency department (ED).

At hospital, a second 12-lead is performed, and a blood sample taken. The 12-lead ECG confirms the prehospital ECG findings. The blood lab work indicates that the troponin I level is elevated at 1.7 ng/ml (normal is < 0.06 ng/ml). The patient is diagnosed with an NSTE-ACS. He is given clopidogrel and a heparin infusion is started. He is then transferred to a cardiac catheter lab where an angiogram is performed showing an 80% occlusion of the proximal right coronary artery and a 90% hazy lesion in the mid-right coronary artery. A stent is placed to reopen the artery and he is discharged 3 days later for follow-up with his cardiologist.

CASE STUDY WRAP-UP

Chest pain is a common complaint for patients with ACS. Although the treatment goal is to reverse the ischemia by improving oxygenation of the injured cardiac tissue, oxygen administration has demonstrated worse outcomes in patients experiencing an ACS when hypoxemia is not present. Oxygen is therefore withheld unless the patient is hypoxic, defined as SaO_2 < 94%, or clinically showing signs of hypoperfusion or dyspnea.

Morphine has also been shown to worsen outcomes in patients experiencing NSTE-ACS. Fentanyl has less of a hemodynamic effect and is felt to be beneficial.

CHAPTER WRAP-UP

Cardiovascular disease is common among elderly Americans and is the leading cause of death in this age group. Early identification of a cardiovascular emergency could reduce mortality and improve recovery times for geriatric patients.

Always consider syncope to be a sign of a life-threatening disorder until proven otherwise. The geriatric age group is susceptible to injury from minor trauma that may have been associated with a syncopal episode.

Prescribed, over-the-counter, and herbal medications can impact the patient's presentation. Clinical findings are further altered by comorbidities and the aging process. Anticipate that the patient will not present as you would expect from younger patients. Ensure any assessment of a geriatric patient is comprehensive and includes a thorough cardiac evaluation.

SS

REFERENCES

American Heart Association. Medications for Arrhythmia. https://www.heart.org/en/health-topics/arrhythmia/prevention--treatment-of-arrhythmia/medications-for-arrhythmia. Published September 30, 2016. Accessed December 11, 2020.

American Heart Association. Types of Blood Pressure Medications. https://www.heart.org/en/health-topics/high-blood-pressure/changes-you-can-make-to-manage-high-blood-pressure/types-of-blood-pressure-medications. Published October 31, 2017. Accessed March 12, 2021.

American Stroke Association. What is a TIA? https://www.stroke.org/en/about-stroke/types-of-stroke/tia-transient-ischemic-attack/what-is-a-tia. Published 2018. Accessed April 16, 2021.

Aroor S, Singh R, Goldstein LB. BE-FAST (Balance, Eyes, Face, Arm, Speech, Time). *Stroke*. 2017;48(2):479–481. doi:10.1161/strokeaha.116.015169

Binning MJ, Sanfillippo G, Rosen W, et al. The neurological emergency room and prehospital stroke alert: the whole is greater than the sum of its parts. *Neurosurgery*. 2014;74(3):281–285; discussion 285. doi:10.1227/NEU.0000000000000259

Buddeke J, Bots ML, Dis I van, et al. Comorbidity in patients with cardiovascular disease in primary care: a cohort study with routine healthcare data. *Br J Gen Pract*. 2019;69(683):e398–e406. doi:10.3399/bjgp19X702725

Centers for Disease Control and Prevention. Types of stroke. https://www.cdc.gov/stroke/types_of_stroke.htm. Updated August 2, 2021. Accessed April 16, 2021.

Crowe F, Zemedikun DT, Okoth K, et al. Comorbidity phenotypes and risk of mortality in patients with ischaemic heart disease in the UK. *Heart*. 2020;106(11):810–816. doi:10.1136/heartjnl-2019-316091

Duncan AK, Vittone J, Fleming KC, Smith HC. *Cardiovascular Disease in Elderly Patients*. Mayo Clinic Proceedings, Symposium on Geriatrics Part VIII. 1996;71(2):184–196.

Francisco AR, Sousa M, Amador P, et al. Chronic medical comorbidities in patients with acute coronary syndrome. *Rev Port Cardiol*. 2010 Jan;29(1):7–21. English, Portuguese. PMID: 20391896.

Fussner J, Velasco C. Stroke Coordinator: Assessing Stroke—Scores & Scales. https://www.stroke.org/-/media/files/affiliates/gra/gra-qsi/2019-scbc-presentations/5--assessing-stroke--scores--scales.pdf. No publication date. Accessed April 16, 2021.

Garcia T. *12-Lead ECG: The Art of Interpretation*. 2nd ed. Burlington, MA: Jones and Bartlett Learning; 2015.

Jackson C, Wenger NK. Cardiovascular disease in the elderly. *Rev Esp Cardiol*. 2011 Aug;64(8):697–712.

Khurshid S, Choi SH, Weng L-C, et al. Frequency of cardiac rhythm abnormalities in a half million adults. *Circ Arrhythm Electrophysiol*. 2018;11(7):e006273. doi:10.1161/CIRCEP.118.006273

Metra M, Zacà V, Parati G, et al. Heart Failure Study Group of the Italian Society of Cardiology. Cardiovascular and noncardiovascular comorbidities in patients with chronic heart failure. *J Cardiovasc Med*. 2011 Feb;12(2):76–84. doi:10.2459/JCM.0b013e32834058d1

National Association of Emergency Medical Technicians. *AMLS: Advanced Medical Life Support: An Assessment-Based Approach*. 3rd ed. Burlington, MA: Jones & Bartlett Learning; 2021.

Pérez de la Ossa N, Carrera D, Gorchs M, et al. Design and validation of a prehospital stroke scale to predict large arterial occlusion. *Stroke*. 2014;45(1):87–91. doi:10.1161/strokeaha.113.003071

Rehman S, Khan A, Rehman A. *Physiology, Coronary Circulation*. StatPearls [Internet]. https://www.ncbi.nlm.nih.gov/books/NBK482413/. Last updated May 2021. Accessed on April 23, 2022.

Salinet ASM, Minhas JS, Panerai RB, Bor-Seng-Shu E, Robinson TG. Do acute stroke patients develop hypocapnia? A systematic review and meta-analysis. *J Neurol Sci*. 2019;402:30–39. doi:10.1016/j.jns.2019.04.038

Virani SS, Alonso A, Benjamin EJ, et al. Heart disease and stroke statistics—2020 update. *Circulation*. 2020;141(9):e139–e596. doi:10.1161/cir.0000000000000757

World Health Organization (WHO). Global health estimates: Leading causes of death. https://www.who.int/data/gho/data/themes/mortality-and-global-health-estimates/ghe-leading-causes-of-death. Published 2019. Accessed March 12, 2021.

World Health Organization (WHO). Hypertension. https://www.who.int/news-room/fact-sheets/detail/hypertension. Published August 25, 2021. Accessed March 12, 2021.

CHAPTER 5

Trauma

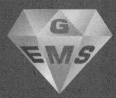

Discuss the relationship between medical conditions and trauma in geriatric patients.

Relate how the changes of aging in body systems may affect trauma incidence, signs and symptoms, complications, and assessment.

Discuss the epidemiology and pathophysiology of the most common traumatic injuries experienced by geriatric patients.

- Identify common geriatric trauma assessment findings using the primary survey and GEMS Diamond.
- Demonstrate the assessment and treatment of geriatric patients suffering the most common geriatric traumas.
- Discuss spinal motion restriction techniques for geriatric patients.

Introduction

As the proportion of elderly in the population increases, so does the incidence of geriatric trauma. Traumatic injuries in the geriatric population present unique challenges in prehospital and hospital care management. Mortality is substantially higher than in younger patients suffering the same injuries. However, evidence shows that geriatric patients are often assessed in the same way as younger patients, resulting in undertriaging the geriatric patient. The physiologic and anatomic changes with age, as well as the patient's baseline health status, must be a component of trauma assessment of the elderly to provide optimal care. The frailty of a geriatric trauma patient has a significant effect on their outcome when trauma occurs.

Handle with Care

Geriatric trauma patients have a higher mortality rate than younger patients regardless of the mechanism of injury.

Trauma is the eighth leading cause of death in patients over the age of 65 years. The most common causes of trauma in older adults are falls, motor vehicle collisions, and burns. Falls account for three-quarters of geriatric trauma and are the most common cause of injury to older adults. Falls are the leading common cause of traumatic death, disability, musculoskeletal injuries, and traumatic brain injuries in older adults. Vehicular trauma and burns are other causes of traumatic injuries that impact the older population differently than in the general younger population. Common traumatic injuries suffered by the older population include traumatic brain injuries, usually caused by falls, cervical and spinal injuries, torso trauma, hip fractures, and extremity injuries.

Aging Changes That Impact Trauma

The aging process affects all body parts and body systems. These changes reflect how the older patient responds differently to trauma than a younger person. Always be aware that what may seem to be a relatively minor injury in an older adult may have severe complications—possibly even life-threatening. Lower your threshold when assessing the mechanism of injury and consider the potential for preexisting conditions when assessing the older patient.

Musculoskeletal Changes

Osteoporosis

Fractures are the most frequent musculoskeletal injuries in the geriatric population. The increased risk of fracture is primarily due to osteoporosis. Osteoporosis is the condition in which normal bone loss exceeds the ability of new bone to be generated to replace it. This causes the bone tissue to become porous and brittle. The weakening of bone structure results in spontaneous fractures, spinal column deformities causing a hunched posture (**FIGURE 5-1**), loss of height, and chronic pain. Common sites of injury associated with osteoporosis are the spinal vertebrae, femur, and radius.

Critical Thinking Question

What other pathologies can occur from immobility due to a musculoskeletal injury?

There is no specific prehospital treatment of osteoporosis. Fractures due to osteoporosis are managed as with fractures in other age groups by providing pain relief and splinting. Medical treatment for osteoporosis can include physiotherapy, calcium and vitamin D supplements, bisphosphonates, monoclonal antibodies, and hormone therapy.

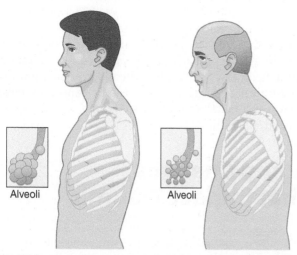

FIGURE 5-1 Spinal curvature can lead to an anteroposterior hump which can cause ventilatory difficulties.

STAR Triad

STAR is an acronym that refers to the most common musculoskeletal disorders affecting the geriatric population: sarcopenia, tendinopathies, and arthritis. These disorders are largely responsible for mobility disorders, pain, increase in fall and fracture risk, and inability to perform activities of daily living.

Sarcopenia involves the loss of muscle mass, strength, and function. This can result from the aging process, an underlying condition, or medication effect. The exact mechanism that causes loss of muscle mass is not understood. Studies have shown that women tend to lose more muscle mass than men.

Symptoms include weakness and an increasingly sedentary lifestyle. The associated decrease in the range of joint motion and strength increases the risk for falls and other injuries. There is no prehospital care for sarcopenia, and medical treatment is limited to exercise and diet counselling.

Gotta Get to the Gym

Studies report a muscle mass decline of 20% in men and 30% in women as we age from 20 to 80 years.

Tendinopathy refers to conditions of tendon pain, swelling, and loss of function during an activity. Symptoms can include tenderness, warmth, swelling, redness, and pain close to the affected tendon. The patient may report stiffness, and crepitus may be noted. It is difficult to differentiate between a tendinopathy and a sprain or fracture without hospital-based diagnostics. Therefore, prehospital care should be limited to pain relief and splinting. Medical treatment focuses on reducing pain of inflammation with anti-inflammatory medication, rest, ice, compression, and elevation.

Arthritis is a disorder of the joints that involves pain, stiffness, reduced range of motion, and swelling. The two most common types are osteoarthritis and rheumatoid arthritis. **Osteoarthritis** is due to cartilage destruction within the joint and is often referred to as a "wear-and-tear" condition. **Rheumatoid arthritis** is much less common and is an autoimmune disease of the joints. It is difficult to differentiate between arthritis and an underlying sprain or fracture without hospital-based diagnostics. Therefore, prehospital care should be limited to pain relief and splinting. Medical treatment includes administration of anti-inflammatories, corticosteroids, and surgery.

Brittle Bones

Osteoarthritis is the most common joint disorder in the world, affecting 80% of adults over the age of 75.

How Cardiovascular Age-Related Changes Impact Trauma

Various age-related cardiovascular changes can affect the geriatric patient:

- Decreased arterial elasticity decreases response to changes in volume status, so there is less compensation for loss of blood, loss of fluid, or volume overload due to aggressive IV therapy.
- Decreased arterial elasticity decreases response to sudden positional changes, which can increase risk of fall when standing up.
- Atherosclerotic changes impair ability to vasoconstrict peripheral vessels, so there is less intravascular shunting and less ability to compensate for blood or fluid loss.
- Preexisting heart failure will impair the ability to compensate for blood or fluid loss.
- Anticoagulant and antiplatelet medications will inhibit clot formation and increase blood loss from hemorrhage.
- Beta blocker medication will inhibit sympathetic response to blood loss so the patient will not compensate, and typical signs and symptoms of shock will not present.

The Heart Grows Weaker with Age

Cardiac output decreases by approximately 50% from ages 20 to 80.

How Respiratory Age-Related Changes Impact Trauma

Respiratory changes can be categorized as involving the airway or breathing. The nasopharyngeal tissues become increasingly fragile with age. Thinning of the nasopharyngeal mucosa increases the risk of bleeding that can be difficult to control and cause aspiration. Changes to the facial bones, skin, and teeth can alter the shape of the face and lead to difficulty in maintaining the airway and providing effective ventilations using a mask. In the lower airways, decreased cilia and decreased cough reflex make it more difficult to clear secretions. There is also an increased risk of rib fractures, clavicle fractures, and flail chest from multiple rib fractures.

How Neurologic Age-Related Changes Impact Trauma

Age-related changes to neurologic function are well known. but are so variable that "normal" aging changes may not be distinguished from pathologic changes. The anticipated "normal" changes include loss of brain tissue mass and neurons. This decrease in brain size creates more volume in the subdural space, which can accommodate blood or swelling in the case of traumatic brain injury and delay the signs and symptoms of increased intracranial pressure. Nerve impulse conduction speed is slower, which can result in small changes in behavior, thinking, and speed of reflexes, leading to an increased risk of falls, fractures, burns, and vehicular trauma.

How Sensory Age-Related Changes Impact Trauma

Vision loss and hearing impairment account for increased risk of the major traumas affecting older adults. Night vision is significantly decreased, so driving at night can be riskier for older drivers. **Peripheral neuropathy** increases the risk for burns and other injuries due to decreased pain sensation. Decreased **psychomotor ability** and impaired balance result in an increased risk of injury from a fall.

Common Mechanisms of Geriatric Injury

Falls

Approximately 33% of adults over 65 years of age experience a fall each year. This increases to 50% by the age of 80 years. Falls typically occur from the standing position to the ground. Causes include deterioration of the musculoskeletal system, which changes posture and gait; decreased vision; deterioration or disorder of the neurologic system, which may cause decreased balance or decreased reflexes; adverse effects of medications; and environmental conditions such as slippery floors, throw rugs, stairs, poorly fitting shoes, poor lighting, and presence of obstacles. Although men and women fall with equal frequency, women are more than twice as likely to sustain a serious injury because of more pronounced osteoporosis. Falls, even those that occur from a standing position, can result in serious injury and life-threatening trauma, with up to 20% to 30% of those who fall sustaining a moderate to severe injury. Long-bone fractures account for the majority of injuries, with fractures of the hip region resulting in the greatest mortality and morbidity rates.

Falls from a moving surface, such as a moving sidewalk or escalator; falls involving stairs; or falls from a height will result in much more complex injuries than expected for a younger adult. Common types of injuries include fractures, soft-tissue wounds, and brain injury ranging from concussion to intracranial hemorrhage.

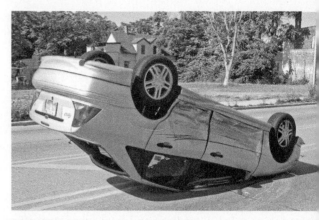

FIGURE 5-2 Rollovers can cause multiple, severe injuries.
© Rechitan Sorin/Shutterstock

Deadly Falls

Falls are the most common cause of traumatic brain injury in older adults.

Immobility caused by a musculoskeletal injury can lead to development of a deep vein thrombosis, pulmonary embolus, skin breakdown leading to pressure sores, sepsis, exposure to infectious pathogens while in the hospital, and loss of independence leading to depression. Death can result from these complications if left untreated.

Victims of a fall may also suffer psychological trauma. After a fall, an older person will typically be more fearful of falling again and may self-isolate or reduce physical activity, which further weakens the body. Ironically, the fear of falling again greatly increases the chances of falling again.

A common call for EMS assistance is the "assist with a lift" complaint involving a patient who has fallen and requires assistance getting up. Such an incident may be due to a serious underlying condition. A thorough assessment of the patient is required to identify the cause of the fall and any injuries. Proper management of this type of call can be lifesaving.

Vehicular Trauma

Motor vehicle collisions (MVCs) are the overall leading cause of trauma deaths globally, and the third leading cause of preventable deaths in the United States (**FIGURE 5-2**). There is an increasing number of older drivers, older vehicle passengers, and older pedestrians due to the increasing geriatric population. When comparing fatalities per mile driven, an increase in fatality rates is seen in drivers starting at ages 70 to 74 years, with the highest rates being among drivers 85 years and older. The older person has an increased risk of being involved in a collision due to slowed reflexes and impaired visual and auditory acuity (**FIGURE 5-3**).

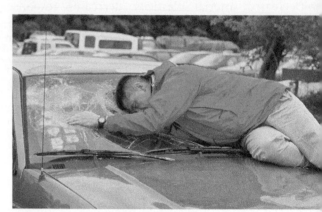

A

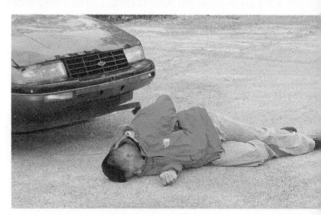

B

FIGURE 5-3 Pedestrian accidents may occur, especially in the geriatric population, due to diminished reflexes and senses.
Copyright © 2024 National Association of Emergency Medical Technicians (NAEMT).

Highest Trauma-Related Mortality

Geriatric patients struck by a vehicle have the highest mortality rate of any age group.

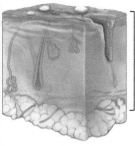

Full thickness
(third degree)
• Leathery
• White to charred
• Dead tissue
• Victims will have pain from burned
  areas adjacent to the full-thickness burn.

FIGURE 5-4 Full thickness burn.

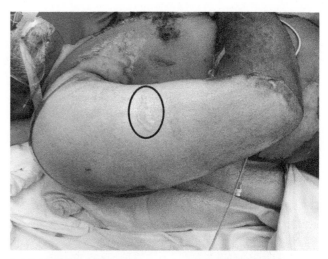

FIGURE 5-5 Partial thickness burns and a full-thickness burn, characterized as white and leathery in appearance.

Courtesy of Dr. Jeffrey Guy

In addition, preexisting conditions such as heart disease, stroke, syncope, and medication effects can suddenly, and without warning, cause the older patient to lose control of a vehicle.

The types of injuries sustained in vehicular trauma are the same as for other age groups. The only exception is that the amount of force required to cause injury is much smaller for older adults. For example, a seatbelt strap may cause bruising or abrasion in a young adult, but the same amount of force may cause a sternal fracture in an older adult.

Burns

Burns have a significantly more damaging effect on older adults than younger patients. Patients age 60 years and older have higher mortality rates for every category of burn severity (**FIGURE 5-4**). A 2001 study showed that age and body surface area burned were the two highest predictors of mortality. Older patients are also more likely to face complications related to burn injuries and subsequent hospitalizations. The top complications include pneumonia, urinary tract infection, and respiratory failure. Unlike in younger patient populations, those age 60 years and older have a greater mortality rate with significantly smaller burn size.

Higher Risk of Death

Mortality is significantly higher for a geriatric patient for any size of burn than a younger adult.

Older adults are more likely to suffer a burn due to various effects of aging (**FIGURE 5-5**). Decreased peripheral sensation and slowed reflexes may cause prolonged contact with a hot surface. Decreased strength and coordination may prevent or slow the escape from scalding water in a bathtub or shower.

Burn treatment for older patients in the hospital is complicated by preexisting disease and impaired functional reserve. In the prehospital setting, these patients are managed the same as younger groups. Transfer to a burn unit is especially recommended for older patients with comorbidities, such as diabetes.

Common Traumatic Injuries in the Geriatric Population

Traumatic Brain Injury

Traumatic brain injury in older adults is associated with higher mortality than the rest of the population. Older adults also have an increased need for long-term care facilities and rehabilitation services. Subdural hematoma is the most frequent traumatic brain injury in older adults.

A **subdural hematoma** usually results from damage to the veins that stretch across the subdural space (**FIGURE 5-6**). When the skull in motion suddenly stops, the brain continues to move within the skull until it hits the interior surface of the skull. The movement of the brain within the skull stretches and tears the veins and bleeding occurs into the subdural space.

Signs and symptoms of the bleeding may not occur for hours, days, or weeks after the injury because the bleeding into the space is slow and, due to brain atrophy in older adults, the subdural space can accommodate a larger amount of blood. A fairly large

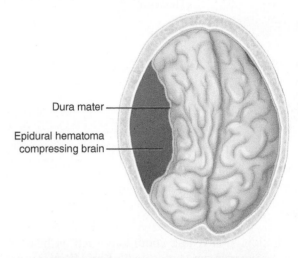

Dura mater

Subdural hematoma
compressing brain

A

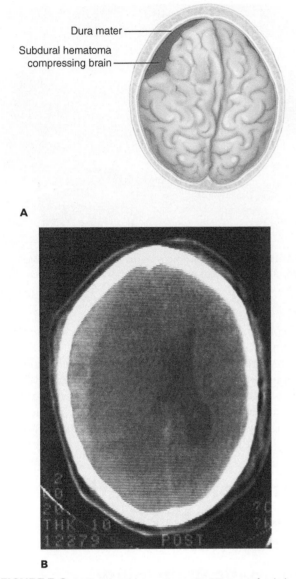

B

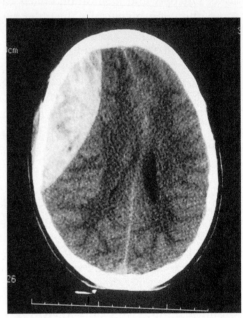

Dura mater

Epidural hematoma
compressing brain

A

B

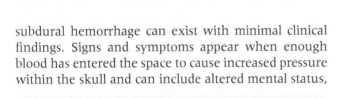

FIGURE 5-6 A. Subdural hematoma. **B.** CT scan of subdural hematoma.

A: Copyright © 2024 National Association of Emergency Medical Technicians (NAEMT). B: Courtesy of Peter T. Pons, MD, FACEP.

FIGURE 5-7 A. Epidural hematoma. **B.** CT scan of epidural hematoma.

A: Copyright © 2024 National Association of Emergency Medical Technicians (NAEMT). B: Courtesy of Peter T. Pons, MD, FACEP.

subdural hemorrhage can exist with minimal clinical findings. Signs and symptoms appear when enough blood has entered the space to cause increased pressure within the skull and can include altered mental status,

Transport to Trauma Center

Patients with suspected skull fracture; penetrating injuries to the head, neck, torso, or proximal extremities; suspected spinal injury with motor or sensory loss; or motor GCS score < 6 should be emergently transported to a trauma center.

unilateral weakness or paralysis on the side opposite the injury, and seizures. A unilaterally dilated pupil on the side of the injury is a late finding. The combination of head trauma and hypovolemic shock yields a greater fatality rate.

Trauma can also cause epidural and subarachnoid hematomas. **Epidural hematoma** involves arterial bleeding into the epidural space due to an artery being torn by a skull fracture (**FIGURE 5-7**). Signs and symptoms appear in minutes to hours and involve a loss of consciousness that can be followed by a temporary lucid period. Other signs and symptoms are the same as for a subdural hematoma.

Subarachnoid hematoma involves blood collecting in the subarachnoid space from an arterial aneurysm rupture. Signs and symptoms of this type of injury will appear suddenly and include sudden, severe headache, nausea and vomiting, and unconsciousness.

Spinal Trauma

The geriatric age group is second only to adolescents and young adults in the number of spinal cord and spinal column injuries. Unlike younger patient groups, spinal cord injury in the geriatric patient tends to be incomplete. This is likely due to less force required to fracture or dislocate the spinal column. Spinal cord injury most often results from hyperextension of the neck. It is also common to have an unstable cervical spinal column fracture after a fall.

Fall Warning: Spinal Injury

Falls are the leading cause of spinal cord and spinal column injury in the geriatric population.

Torso Trauma

The high rate of mortality from motor vehicle collisions is due to the high number of chest injuries sustained in this type of trauma. Thoracic trauma from an MVC is the second leading cause of traumatic death after brain injury. Chest injuries, such as a fractured rib, can exacerbate preexisting cardiopulmonary conditions, which can be life-threatening. Rib fractures, flail chest, and lung contusion will further impair breathing due to pain and, in the case of flail chest, loss of mechanical function of the ribs. Injury to the lung tissue will further increase airway resistance and may imitate a pneumothorax presentation.

Traumatic aortic disruption is also a frequent injury because the aorta is prone to damage due to increased stiffness and dilation caused by age-related changes. Signs and symptoms of this type of injury are nonspecific and therefore unreliable. Thus, assessment of aortic disruption hinges on index of suspicion. A high index should be maintained in situations involving high-energy deceleration/acceleration mechanisms. The prehospital care practitioner needs to assess the adequacy of the airway and breathing and should carefully auscultate and palpate the chest. Careful examination may demonstrate that the pulse quality may be different between the two upper extremities (pulse stronger in the right arm than the left) or between the upper (brachial artery) and lower extremities (femoral artery). Blood pressures, if measured, may be higher in the upper extremities than in the lower extremities, comprising the signs of a pseudo-coarctation (narrowing) of the aorta.

Beware the Lack of Signs and Symptoms

Fifty percent of geriatric patients with an aortic injury appear uninjured.

Hip Fracture

In the United States, there are approximately 350,000 hip fractures each year—the second leading cause of hospitalization of geriatric patients. Hip fracture subsets include femoral head fracture and **proximal femoral fracture**, which includes femoral neck fracture.

Femoral head fractures are almost always due to a traumatic hip dislocation. Treatment is urgent and requires the reduction of the dislocated hip under anesthesia. **Femoral neck fractures** make up about 90% of proximal femoral fractures. They are the most common kind of hip fractures.

A Cause of Permanent Disability and Death

Femoral neck fractures often result in permanent disability and can result in death within the first year, postinjury, for up to 33% of patients.

Extremity Injuries

Lower extremity injuries in the older population are usually due to knee stiffness, osteoporosis-related bone fragility, and medial rotation of the ankle. Common mechanisms include misjudging the height of a step or forcefully depressing a brake pedal.

Falls are the most common frequent mechanism for upper extremity injuries. Shoulders and wrists are the usual sites of injury.

Trauma Assessment of the Geriatric Patient
GEMS Diamond in Trauma

The GEMS Diamond should be applied in any trauma injury in a geriatric patient. The G in GEMS is a reminder that geriatric patients can present atypically.

Also, keep in mind that traumatic injuries are more likely to cause serious repercussions for older patients, including loss of independence, so always treat older patients with dignity and respect, and be mindful of their concerns.

Trauma is most often related to the patient's environment, so let the E in GEMS remind you to assess for the cause of trauma such as rugs, slippery floor surfaces, uneven floors or stairs, poor lighting, broken or unused assistive devices, and obstacles that may act as potential trip hazards. EMS personnel are often the only medical practitioners to have access to a patient's living conditions; prevention is the best approach, so assess for the potential for trauma when you are responding to a medical complaint.

Traumatic injuries can have a medical component, so the M in GEMS reminds you to obtain a thorough medical history, including all medications taken.

The S in GEMS should remind you to assess the patient's social conditions with respect to the possibility of abuse, as the cause of trauma. Social support should also be considered for patients who have suffered a fall and need support for optimal recovery. Include your concerns as part of your patient care report so that arrangements can be made for increased support when the patient is discharged from hospital.

Scene Assessment

As always, the initial concern when approaching a scene is for the safety for yourself, your coresponders, bystanders, and the patient. However, safety issues for a geriatric patient are different than those for a younger adult. For instance, walking on uneven ground in darkness may pose little risk to a young person but significant risk to an older adult. When evaluating safety concerns for a geriatric patient, you must consider the scene from their perspective.

Often, the clues to the mechanism of injury are subtle, and less energy is required to cause injury. You may find that mechanism of injury does not match the severity of the patient's condition. A preexisting condition also may play a part in the patient's clinical presentation, creating a combination of medical and traumatic complaints. The incidence of chronic medical conditions increases with age; thus, an older adult is more likely to suffer trauma as the consequence of a medical problem than a younger adult. For instance, a seat-belted geriatric patient may be in cardiac arrest following or preceding a low-impact "fender-bender" motor vehicle collision.

Include bystander feedback in your scene assessment, which may include a report that the patient appeared unconscious prior to a collision. A medical ID bracelet may indicate an underlying chronic condition.

The information from your scene assessment is important to share with the receiving facility.

As with incidents involving any age of patients, evaluate the scene for the need of additional resources. Unlike scenes involving other patients, place emphasis on ambient temperature, as geriatric patients are less able to tolerate both hot and cold environments and more easily suffer hyper- or hypothermia. Protecting the patient from the environment may be a higher priority when managing the care of an older patient.

> **Fragile—Handle with Care**
>
> Geriatric patients' bodies are much more fragile than younger patients. A minor mechanism of injury can cause significant injury.

Primary Survey

Preexisting conditions, medications, and age-related changes complicate the clinical findings associated with trauma. Pain may be masked by age-related deterioration of the sensory neurons or pain-blocking effects of medication for chronic pain. Some older patients develop an increased tolerance to pain and may not complain to the same degree as a younger patient. A thorough hands-on physical examination of the patient is necessary to properly locate all injuries (**TABLE 5-1**).

Multiple injured sites in various degrees of healing may be found. This could be the result of multiple traumatic incidents such as repeated falls, especially if the patient is confused or weakened by malnourishment or dehydration. Multiple traumas, malnourishment, or dehydration could be signs of elder abuse. Collecting a complete history, including social support, will aid in appropriately managing such cases.

SPLATT Assessment

SPLATT is a mnemonic used during a post-fall assessment to help prevent future falls (**TABLE 5-2**).

Presentation and Timing of Symptoms

Typical findings of serious illness such as fever, pain, or tenderness may take longer to develop in the older patient and can delay or temporarily hide the presenting signs and symptoms. Pain perception may also be affected. Due to the normal aging process and the presence of neuropathies from diseases such as diabetes, some older adults may perceive pain differently than patients who have not experienced chronic pain. This

TABLE 5-1 Factors That Can Alter the Significance of Assessment Findings

	General impression	Mechanism of injury may not be apparent. Patient will present atypically and may even appear uninjured.
X	Exsanguinating bleed	Anticoagulant medications interfere with normal clotting process, so bleeding is more persistent.
A	Airway	Decreased cough reflex and anticoagulant medication can increase risk of aspiration.
B	Breathing	Rib fracture pain may be tolerated better than younger patients. Diminished surface for gas exchange makes oxygenation more difficult. Increased airway pressure can complicate effective ventilation.
C	Circulation	Medications may mask pain and sympathetic response. Blood vessels are weakened and are easily damaged.
D	Disability	Altered mentation and lower GCS score may be normal baseline for older patients. Pupils may not be able to be assessed due to cataract surgery scarring.
E	Expose/ environment	Decreased temperature tolerance makes geriatric patients more prone to hypothermia.

Copyright © 2024 National Association of Emergency Medical Technicians (NAEMT).

TABLE 5-2 SPLATT Assessment

Mnemonic	Assessment
S	Symptoms the patient had prior to the fall could identify a medical disorder which led to the fall.
P	Previous falls suffered by the patient could identify a pattern of cause.
L	Location of fall could identify hazards that caused the fall.
A	Activity immediately prior to fall could identify need for assist devices or other form of support.
T	Time of day could identify need for better lighting.
T	Trauma that caused or resulted from the fall that can be corrected (could be physical or psychological)

Copyright © 2024 National Association of Emergency Medical Technicians (NAEMT).

perception places them at increased risk of injury from burns or excesses in heat and cold exposure.

Living with daily pain can cause an increased tolerance to pain, which may result in a patient's failure to identify areas of injury. When evaluating patients with traumatic injuries, especially those who regularly experience diffuse body pain or who appear to have a high tolerance to pain, prehospital care practitioners should identify areas in which the pain has increased in intensity or in which the painful area has enlarged.

Note the pain characteristics or exacerbating factors since the trauma occurred. A good mnemonic to capture this information is OPQRST. Previous injuries may cause weakness in the injured area, which can increase the risk of a repeat injury.

Geriatric Trauma Care Tips

Temperature Management

Older patients are at an increased risk for hypothermia and hyperthermia due to age-related changes impairing their ability to maintain normal body heat. This can be of concern during periods of prolonged extrication from the scene. External warming and cooling measures should be implemented (**FIGURE 5-8**). A sheet or patient clothing should be used as a barrier between the heating or cooling source and the patient's skin to prevent iatrogenic injury. Minimize skin exposure during physical examination. Recall that certain medications for Parkinson disease, depression, psychosis, and nausea can make a patient more prone to overheating.

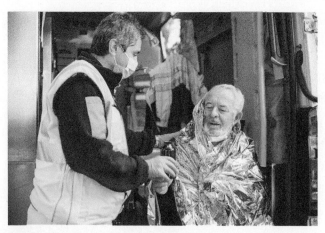

FIGURE 5-8 Remember that older patients are at an increased risk for hypothermia and hyperthermia and attention should be paid to maintaining their normal body heat at all times.

© loreanto/Shutterstock

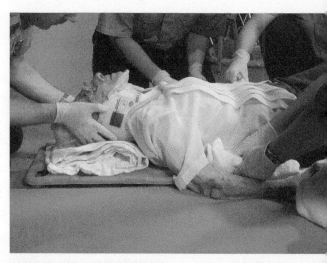

FIGURE 5-9 Immobilization of a kyphotic patient.

© Jones & Bartlett Learning

Spinal Motion Restriction

Spinal motion restriction follows the same application principles as for younger patients in that protecting the cervical, thoracic, and lumbar spine in a patient who has sustained multisystem trauma is the standard of care.

Degenerative arthritis of the cervical spine can cause a spinal cord injury to occur during positioning and manipulating the neck while managing the airway. Practitioners should know and follow their local protocols for patient stabilization and spinal motion restriction.

Severe kyphosis, an osteoporosis-related hunching of the spinal column, may create additional complications if a cervical collar is applied. Practitioners should ensure that if used, the collar does not inadvertently compress the airway or carotid arteries. Alternative methods using a rolled towel and head block may be necessary. In a supine older patient with kyphosis, extra padding, such as a blanket or dressings, may be required to reduce pressure on bony prominences if rigid splinting is used (**FIGURE 5-9**). For these patients a vacuum mattress may provide appropriate support and greater comfort.

NSAIDS is a mnemonic that can be used to recall considerations for spinal motion restriction (**TABLE 5-3**).

Cardiovascular Considerations

Decreasing ability of the cardiovascular system to compensate for blood or fluid loss means that shock will progress quickly from the initial injury to a refractory state of shock and death. Assessment of cardiac trauma is limited in the prehospital setting. Prompt recognition of an impending or progressing shock state requires rapid transport to a trauma center.

TABLE 5-3 NSAIDS: Considerations for Spinal Motion Restriction

Mnemonic	Considerations for Spinal Motion Restriction
N	Neurologic—presence of a focal or neurologic deficit
S	Significant mechanism of injury—high likelihood of spinal column instability due to force of injury
A	Altered mental status—patient is an unreliable historian
I	Intoxication
D	Distracting injury—patient has an injury painful enough to distract them from the pain of a neck injury or spinal tenderness
S	Spinal tenderness—signs or symptoms of injury apparent

Copyright © 2024 National Association of Emergency Medical Technicians (NAEMT).

Respiratory Considerations

Treatment of respiratory system trauma in a geriatric patient should include prompt provision of supplemental oxygen. Rib injuries are self-splinted by the patient. If breathing is impaired and inadequate, provide positive-pressure ventilations with oxygen. Placement of an advanced airway will be required if higher airway pressures prevent effective positive-pressure ventilation. Needle decompression is indicated when a tension pneumothorax is suspected.

Decreased chest wall elasticity can lead to increased positive-pressure ventilation pressures and gastric inflation. Gastric inflation, in turn, further decreases chest expansion by putting pressure on the diaphragm and increases the risk of vomiting with consequent aspiration. Decreased chest wall movement and decreased alveolar surface mean less opportunity for gas exchange when it is needed the most.

CASE STUDY

It is 0800 on a warm spring morning. You and your partner are staffing an emergency response ambulance and are dispatched to a single-family suburban house for an 80-year-old female who is confused (**FIGURE 5-10**).

QUESTIONS

- What is your differential diagnosis?
  - AMS is a nonspecific complaint and can be seen in numerous conditions, so without additional information, it is almost impossible to narrow down the options. Differential diagnosis should be reconsidered once the primary assessment is complete and you have more information with which to work.
- How does the patient's age affect your assessment approach?
  - Include the GEMS Diamond as part of your overall assessment.

The area appears safe as you don your PPE while approaching the house. You are met at the door by the patient's daughter. She takes you to her mother, who is sitting in a recliner in the living room. The scene appears safe. As you approach the patient, your initial impression is that she is alert, her breathing is normal, and her skin color is good. The house is well-kept, warm, obstacle-free, and there is plenty of light. The patient is appropriately dressed and has no glasses, hearing aids, or walking assists. You also notice a small hematoma to the right forehead and a skin tear with bruising to her right arm.

The daughter tells you that her mother lives with her. She states that yesterday her mother fell on the bathroom floor when she tripped on a rug while getting out of the shower. She heard her mother fall and when she got to the bathroom, she found her mother conscious and lying on the floor. She did not appear to have hit anything while falling. She assisted her mother to her feet and helped her get dressed. She bandaged the skin tear and asked her mother if she wanted to see a doctor. Her mother adamantly refused medical attention. Her mother seemed fine until today.

The daughter said she called EMS this morning because her mother is confused and not acting normally since waking about an hour ago. Her mother felt fine and did not appear to be confused yesterday.

QUESTIONS

- What could have caused the patient to fall (remember that it was unwitnessed)?
  - The daughter reported that her mother tripped over a rug, but it is important to consider other causes that could have affected the patient's balance (syncope, medication effects, musculoskeletal/ cardiovascular/neurologic conditions).

- Do you have any concerns based on your initial impression?
  - AMS is always a concern, especially in patients who are otherwise fully oriented.

You perform a primary survey:

- X–No significant external bleeding
- A–Airway is patent
- B–Breathing is regular and normal depth, lung sounds are clear and equal bilaterally
- C–Radial pulses are strong and irregular, skin is warm, dry, and normal color
- D–GCS 13 (E4, V3, M6), she is confused to place and time, has no recollection of her fall yesterday, her speech consists of inappropriate words, pupils are equal in size but right pupil has a sluggish response to light

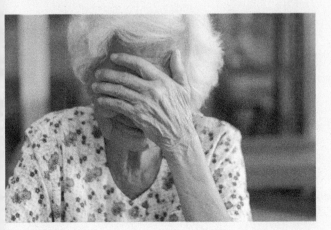

FIGURE 5-10

- E–2-inch (5 cm) skin tear and purple-colored bruising to the right arm, 1 inch (2.5 cm) diameter hematoma to right forehead, no edema, no rashes

QUESTIONS

- What is the cardinal presentation and the chief complaint?
  - Cardinal presentation is altered mental status. Chief complaint is difficult to assess given the patient's AMS and difficulty communicating.

- Are any interventions required before assessment can continue?
  - No interventions are required at this time.

- Does this patient require immediate transport, or can you remain on scene and continue your assessment?
  - At present, the patient is stable enough to continue your assessment on scene.

- What further assessments would you like to perform?
  - Given the patient's age and symptoms, a stroke assessment would be warranted.

You attempt to obtain a patient history using the OPQRST mnemonic, but the patient is unable to provide much information:

- O–Onset is unknown as it occurred sometime in the night before waking
- P–Unknown
- Q–Unknown
- R–Unknown
- S–Unknown
- T–1 hour

The SAMPLER history is collected from the daughter as the patient is unable to communicate.

- S–AMS, confusion
- A–No known allergies
- M–Aspirin, apixaban, metoprolol, and diltiazem
- P–Atrial fibrillation and hypertension
- L–A piece of toast this morning
- E–Unwitnessed fall yesterday and unable to recall fall
- R–Age, apixaban prescription will inhibit clotting

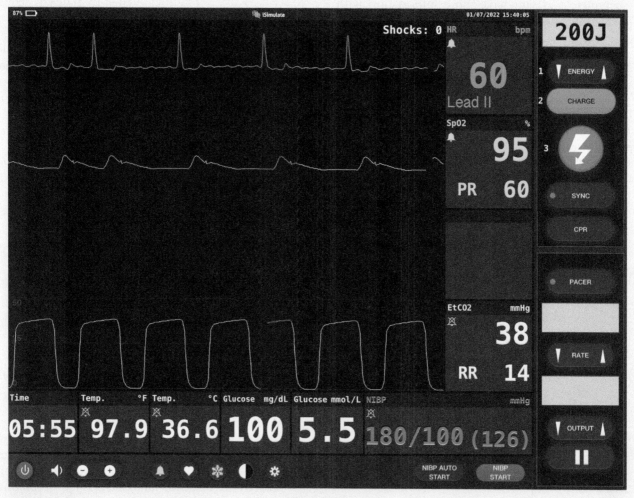

FIGURE 5-11

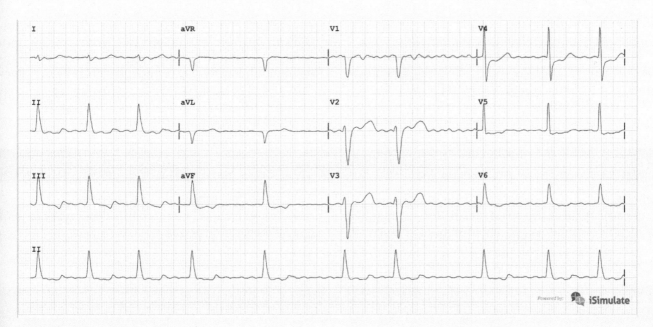

FIGURE 5-12

You perform a stroke assessment and find that she has no arm drift, her smile is equal; and, although she uses the wrong words, her speech is clear. With this assessment, you rule out stroke.

You further assess the patient by measuring her blood pressure and attaching a cardiac monitor and oximeter. The results of these assessments are as follows:

- HR: 60, irregular
- BP: 180/100

- RR: 14
- Temp: 97.9°F (36.6°C) tympanic
- SpO$_2$: 95% on room air
- ETCO$_2$: 38 mm Hg
- ECG: atrial fibrillation

A 12-lead ECG shows indeterminant ST changes, and BGL is 100 mg/dl (5.5 mmol/L). A brief head-to-toe examination reveals no new findings or signs of trauma.

GEMS DIAMOND REVIEW

How was the GEMS Diamond information applied in this case?

 Geriatric Assessment: The patient is an 80-year-old female. She has impaired hearing, two comorbidities, four prescriptions, and does not use hearing aids, glasses, or walking assists.

 Environmental Assessment: The home is well maintained, rug in bathroom is a possible trip hazard, hand grips may be needed to exit shower safely.

 Medical Assessment: Patient is compliant with prescriptions; anticoagulant prescription could lead to serious internal bleeding.

 Social Assessment: Patient is independent and performs ADLs independently, daughter and son-in-law provide extra support with meal preparations and medication administration.

QUESTIONS

- Where should this patient be transported?
  - This patient should be transported to the closest facility with neurologic capabilities.

- What other assessments are likely to be performed in the hospital?
  - Given the potential for head injury (as evidenced by the hematoma), CT scan of the head will be likely to check for intracranial bleeding. Monitoring of anticoagulant medications may also be performed to reduce the risk of additional bleeding.

- What else can be done for this patient beyond her immediate medical care?
  - An environmental assessment should be performed to check for hazards and improve the patient's safety.

The patient is placed on a stretcher in a position of comfort and transported to the closest facility with a CT scanner and neurology department. The head of the stretcher is elevated 30 degrees and intravenous access is established using a saline lock injection site.

There are no changes en route to the hospital. At the hospital, a CT scan reveals a subdural hematoma. Given the patient's age and comorbidities, a conservative approach to her care is decided upon and surgical drainage of the hematoma is not performed. Her

antiplatelet and anticoagulant therapies are discontinued, and she is admitted to the neurologic unit. After 3 days in the hospital, she is transferred to a rehabilitation facility where she recovers fully. A home-care assessment recommends removal of throw rugs in the home and placement of strategically placed handholds to prevent further falls.

CASE STUDY WRAP-UP

Falls are not to be taken lightly when responding to a geriatric patient. Hospital evaluation is required to identify or rule out potential injuries. Prevention

through proper follow-up and environmental assessment is also a critical piece to the overall management of a fallen geriatric person.

CHAPTER WRAP-UP

Falls are the leading cause of injury and death due to trauma in the geriatric population. Fractures are the most frequent musculoskeletal injuries among older adults, primarily due to falls and osteoporosis.

Incorporating the GEMS Diamond into your geriatric trauma assessment will assist in identifying hazards commonly associated with falls, burns, vehicular trauma, and other injuries.

REFERENCES

Abdelmalik PA, Draghic N, Ling GSF. Management of moderate and severe traumatic brain injury. *Transfusion*. 2019;59(S2): 1529–1538. doi:10.1111/trf.15171

Adams SD, Holcomb JB. Geriatric trauma. *Curr Opin Crit Care*. 2015;21(6):520–526.

Arden A, Nevitt M. Osteoarthritis: epidemiology. *Best Pract Res Clin Rheumatol*. 2006;20(1):3–25.

Caterino JM, Brown NV, Hamilton MW, et al. Effect of geriatric-specific trauma triage criteria on outcomes in injured older adults: a statewide retrospective cohort study. *J Am Geriatr Soc*. 2016;64(10):1944–1951.

Choi K, Jeon G, Cho S. Prospective study on the impact of fear of falling on functional decline among community dwelling elderly women. *Int J Environ Res Public Health*. 2017;14(5):469. doi:10.3390/ijerph14050469

Centers for Disease Control and Prevention. Important Facts about Falls. https://www.cdc.gov/homeandrecreationalsafety/falls /adultfalls.html. Published 2019. Accessed February 14, 2021.

Colwell C. Geriatric trauma: Initial evaluation and management. https://www.uptodate.com/contents/geriatric-trauma-initial -evaluation-and-management/print. Updated July 16, 2021. Accessed March 23, 2021.

Gheno R, Cepparo JM, Rosca CE, Cotten A. Musculoskeletal disorders in the elderly. *J Clin Imaging Sci*. 2012;2(1):39. doi:10.4103/2156-7514.99151

Giordano V, Giordano M, Glória RC, et al. General principles for treatment of femoral head fractures. *J Clin Orthop Trauma*. 2019;10(1):155–160. doi:10.1016/j.jcot.2017.07.013

Hashmi A, Ibrahim-Zada I, Rhee P, et al. Predictors of mortality in geriatric patients: a systematic review and meta-analysis. *J Trauma Acute Care Surg*. 2014;76(3):894–901.

Institute of Medicine (US) Division of Health Promotion and Disease Prevention; Berg RL, Cassells JS, eds. *The Second Fifty Years: Promoting Health and Preventing Disability*. Washington, DC: National Academies Press; 1992:15, Falls in older persons: risk factors and prevention. https://www.ncbi.nlm.nih.gov/books /NBK235613/

Jacobs DG. Special considerations in geriatric injury. *Curr Opin Crit Care*. 2003;9(6):535–539.

Joseph B, Hassan A. Geriatric trauma patients: what is the difference? *Cur Surg Rep*. 2015;4(1). doi:10.1007/s40137 -015-0123-0

Landers MR, Oscar S, Sasaoka J, Vaughn K. Balance confidence and fear of falling avoidance behavior are most predictive of falling in older adults: prospective analysis. *Phys Ther*. 2016;96(4):433–442.

Mayo Clinic. Osteoporosis. https://www.mayoclinic.org/diseases -conditions/osteoporosis/symptoms-causes/syc-20351968. Published August 21, 2021. Accessed March 1, 2021.

Minetto MA, Giannini A, McConnell R, Busso C, Torre G, Massazza G. Common musculoskeletal disorders in the elderly: the STAR triad. *J Clin Med*. 2020;9(4):1216. doi:10.3390/jcm9041216

Mohta M, Sethi AK, Tyagi A, Mohta A. Psychological care in trauma patients. *Injury*. 2003;34(1):17–25. doi:10.1016/s0020-1383(02) 00377-7

Morris J, McManus D. The neurology of aging: normal versus pathologic change. *Geriatrics*. 1991;46(8):47–48, 51–54.

Murphy SL, Xu J, Kochanek KD, Arias E, Tejada-Vera B. Deaths: final data for 2018. *National Vital Statistics Reports*. 2021;69(13). https://www.cdc.gov/nchs/data/nvsr/nvsr69/nvsr69-13-508.pdf. Published January 12, 2021. Accessed February 14, 2021.

National Association of Emergency Medical Technicians. *PHTLS: Prehospital Trauma Life Support*. 9th ed. Burlington, MA: Jones & Bartlett Learning; 2020.

National Fire Protection Association. Characteristics of home fire victims. 2014. https://www.nfpa.org/News-and-Research/Fire-statistics-and-reports/Fire-statistics/Demographics-and-victim-patterns/Characteristics-of-home-fire-victims

Southern AP, Lopez RA, Jwayyed S. Geriatric trauma. In: StatPearls [Internet]. https://www.ncbi.nlm.nih.gov/books/NBK442020/. Updated 2022 Jul 18. Accessed April 10, 2022.

Wibbenmeyer LA, Amelon MJ, Morgan LJ, et al. Predicting survival in an elderly burn patient population. *Burns*. 2001 Sep;27(6):583–590. doi:10.1016/s0305-4179(01)00009-2

Zhao F, Tang B, Hu C, Wang B, Wang Y, Zhang L. The impact of frailty on posttraumatic outcomes in older trauma patients: a systematic review and meta-analysis. *J Trauma Acute Care Surg*. 2020 April;88(4):546–554.

CHAPTER 6

Other Medical Disorders

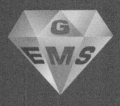

- Recognize the impact of age-related changes to the geriatric patient's gastrointestinal, renal, genitourinary, and endocrine systems.
- Identify causes of abdominal pain, including common gastrointestinal, renal, genitourinary, and endocrine disorders in geriatric patients.

- Discuss the pathophysiology of gastrointestinal, renal, genitourinary, and endocrine disorders.
- Identify other common medical emergencies in the older adult.
- Apply assessment and management strategies to a geriatric patient with renal failure.

Challenges Associated with Abdominal Pain in the Older Adult

Abdominal pain can be a challenging complaint to diagnose for any age of patient. This complaint is further complicated for geriatric patients due to age-related changes, comorbidities, and medications. These factors can cause a delay in the onset of signs and symptoms, produce unexpected physical findings, or result in variable vital signs. Often, the geriatric patient will not present with "textbook" clinical features. Instead, patients will present much later in the course of their illness and have nonspecific complaints. For instance, the vague complaint of generalized weakness may be due to an abdominal disorder.

A Common Problem

Abdominal pain is one of the most common geriatric patient entrance complaints to the emergency department (ED).

Due to the complex nature of an abdominal pain complaint, a broader differential diagnosis must be considered.

This means that more diagnostic studies are needed, resulting in prolonged stays in the ED. Additionally, geriatric patients with abdominal pain are much more likely to be admitted to the hospital or require surgery. Early identification and management of the pain source, even in the prehospital setting, can improve patient outcomes. A routine prehospital physical examination can appear to be normal even if a lethal condition, such as abdominal aortic aneurysm rupture or mesenteric ischemia, is present. Even the slightest abdominal complaint by older adult patient must be taken very seriously.

Added Complications

Polypharmacy adds to the complications with gastrointestinal (GI) symptoms due to adverse effects from drug interactions or drug effects on a preexisting condition.

Gastrointestinal System Changes with Age

Changes to the upper gastrointestinal (GI) tract due to age put the older adult patient at increased risk of aspiration and malnutrition (TABLE 6-1). These changes include more difficult chewing due to dental issues,

TABLE 6-1 Age-Related Changes to GI Tract and Abdominal Pain

Age-Related Change	Source of Pain
Decreased blood flow to GI tract	Pain due to ischemic tissues
Decreased ability to resist damage to lining of the stomach	Increased risk for peptic ulcers
Decreased tongue and esophageal muscle strength	Increased risk of aspiration
Slowed motility of the GI tract, decreased blood flow to the intestines and liver	Increased risk of acid reflux, constipation, and bowel obstruction; decreased ability to metabolize substances
Weakening of anal sphincter muscles	Stool incontinence
Increased incidence of constipation, physical inactivity, and decreased immune function	Increased risk for development of diverticulitis
Decreased blood flow to the gallbladder, poor diet and inactivity, medication effect, and decreased immune function	Increased risk of developing cholecystitis
Medication use, cholecystitis, and alcohol consumption	Increased risk of pancreatitis

decreased salivation to moisten chewed food, decreased tongue and esophageal muscle strength, decreased gag reflex, and decreased cough reflex. Older adults may eat less frequently or consume smaller amounts of food out of fear of choking, which can result in malnutrition.

With age, there is a decrease in absorption of nutrients and other substances in the intestines, which can also lead to malnutrition. Accessory organs are affected as well. The liver has a reduced ability to metabolize toxins and medications.

Abdominal pain can also result from non-GI conditions. Heart failure (HF) can cause abdominal ischemia due to decreased systolic blood flow to the abdomen and hepatic congestion as cardiac preload increases. Atrial fibrillation (A-fib) is correlated with embolic events, which can cause abdominal pain due to ischemia. Atherosclerosis can lead to myocardial infarction that may present with abdominal discomfort. It may also cause an abdominal aortic aneurysm, which can present with abdominal pain when rupturing or dissecting. Other non-GI causes of abdominal pain can include pneumonia, hypercalcemia, and shingles.

Poor Outcomes

Morbidity and mortality are high among geriatric patients complaining of abdominal pain.

Renal System Changes with Age

Significant loss of kidney mass occurs with aging. In addition to the loss of nephrons, there is a decrease in the autoregulation of blood flow and renal filtration functions. Decreased renal perfusion results from vascular volume depletion, HF, and hypotension. **Nephrotoxins**, such as certain medications, can lead to acute tubular necrosis. Necrosis can also result from rhabdomyolysis, a byproduct of muscle tissue breakdown, and administration of medical contrast dye.

Kidney Dysfunction

Kidney function decreases approximately 50% between the ages of 20 and 90 years.

The reduction in blood flow to the kidneys means that the filtration required to produce urine also slows. Because of the slower rate of filtration, not all waste products and toxins are excreted. The decreased ability to excrete drugs from the bloodstream means medication levels in the blood can slowly increase to toxic levels or interact with other medications. The leading cause of drug interaction problems in older patients is an underlying renal dysfunction.

Genitourinary System Changes with Age

Along with the kidneys, the urinary bladder also gets smaller. Since urine is continuously being produced, the reduced urinary bladder size means there is less ability to delay urination after first sensing the need to urinate. Sporadic contractions of the urinary bladder walls and postmenopausal changes to the bladder and urethra also decrease the ability to control urination, making incontinence common in older adults, especially women.

Urination can become difficult with age due to weakening of the muscles in the urinary bladder walls and the enlargement of the prostate in men, which can obstruct flow through the urethra. Incomplete emptying of the bladder can lead to more frequent urination and increased risk of urinary tract infection. Obstruction of urine flow or untreated infection can lead to kidney damage and a further decrease of kidney function.

Endocrine System Changes with Age

Because hormones control the body, a decline of hormone production will affect an older person systemically. For example, a decrease in thyroid hormone will affect red blood cell production, causing the person to become anemic and complain of general fatigue. That same decrease will also affect glucose control and muscle mass. The thyroid gland secretes the hormones tetraiodothyronine (T4) and triiodothyronine (T3), which are responsible for regulating the body's vital signs.

Metabolic changes increase the risk of type 2 diabetes, stroke, and hypertension. Weight gain and obesity impact mobility and increase the risk of falls.

Gastrointestinal Disorders and Abdominal Pain

Gastroesophageal Reflux Disease

Gastroesophageal reflux disease (GERD) occurs when stomach contents move up past the lower esophageal sphincter into the esophagus. The esophagus does not have the same protective lining as the stomach, so the acidic stomach contents irritate the esophageal walls and cause pain. Many medications will increase the risk of GERD in geriatric patients.

Not Doing So GERD

GERD is the most common GI disorder in older adults, affecting 23% of the geriatric population.

Signs and symptoms of GERD include difficulty swallowing, vomiting, heartburn, acid regurgitation into the esophagus, and difficulty breathing. Prehospital care is supportive and may include pain relief.

GERD is treated with prescriptions of proton pump inhibitors or bicarbonate mineral water hydration to lower stomach acidity, or prokinetic drugs to speed passage of food through the stomach. Management may also include dietary changes, such as reducing food portions or not eating late at night.

Silent Reflux

Silent reflux, or laryngopharyngeal reflux (LPR), has the same pathology as GERD, but does not have the classic GERD symptoms. Typical GERD symptoms are not present. LPR symptoms include post-nasal drip, dry cough, hoarseness, and the feeling of a "lump" in the throat.

Silent reflux can be hard to diagnose due to atypical presentation, and patients may confuse symptoms with an upper respiratory infection, allergies, or another pathology.

Peptic Ulcer Disease

Peptic ulcer disease (PUD) involves a breakdown of duodenal or gastric mucosa and subsequent damage to tissues by stomach acid (**FIGURE 6-1**). PUD can be caused by long-term use of nonsteroidal anti-inflammatory drugs (NSAIDs), which block the chemical protection of the gastric lining; *Helicobacter pylori* infection, which

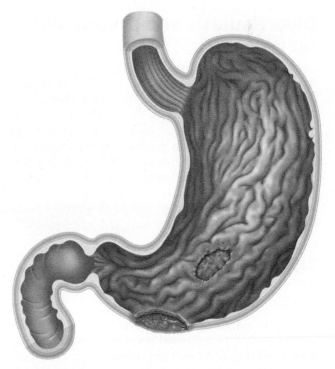

FIGURE 6-1 Gastric ulcers caused by peptic ulcer disease.
© ilusmedical/Shutterstock

directly damages the mucosal lining; and tumors that increase stomach acidity. Polypharmacy has also been linked to an increased risk of PUD. Medications involved include oral steroids, anticoagulants, and selective serotonin reuptake inhibitors (SSRIs).

Vomiting Blood Is Likely PUD

PUD is the most common cause of upper GI bleeding in geriatric patients.

PUD symptoms in geriatric patients differ from younger patients. Signs and symptoms include "burning" stomach pain, feeling of bloating, heartburn, and nausea. The most common severe sign is melena, or black and tarry stool. Only about one-third of geriatric patients report epigastric pain. This lack of pain often delays diagnosis, which can lead to pyloric stenosis, more severe hemorrhage, and perforation. Signs of severe bleeding include vomiting blood, feeling faint, and trouble breathing. If the ulcer is allowed to erode to perforation, free air will enter the abdomen and sepsis will ultimately occur.

Prehospital management of this type of patient involves protection of the airway from aspiration, ensuring adequate oxygenation, possibly offering pain relief, and treating hypovolemia if present. Hospital care focuses on pain relief, infection control, and addressing risk factors such as reducing NSAID use, increasing dietary fiber, and relieving constipation.

Diverticulosis and Diverticulitis

After the age of 40 years, small bulging pouches called **diverticula** can form in the weaker areas of the intestinal lining, especially in the colon (**FIGURE 6-2**). **Diverticulosis** is the condition in which these diverticula exist. **Diverticulitis** is the condition in which inflammation and infection occurs in one or more diverticula. Diverticulosis is generally asymptomatic, but can cause abdominal tenderness, cramping, bloating, **hematochezia** (red blood in the stool), or constipation.

The Colon Gets Pouchy with Age

In the United States, half the population over the age of 60 have diverticulosis, and that number increases to 65% by age 85.

Diverticulitis is thought to occur when the diverticula erode due to increased pressure or become filled with stool that is pushed into them. Signs and symptoms of diverticulitis include pain or tenderness at the lower left quadrant, fever, nausea and vomiting, chills, cramps, constipation or diarrhea, and hematochezia.

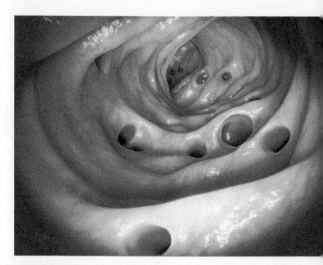

FIGURE 6-2 Diverticula present in the large intestine.
© Juan Gaertner/Shutterstock

Prehospital care is supportive and may include pain relief, although practitioners should assess and treat hypovolemia from GI bleeding if present. Medical care includes maintaining adequate oxygenation, pain management, infection control, and reducing risk factors such as NSAID use, lack of dietary fiber, and constipation.

Constipation and Fecal Incontinence

Constipation is generally described as chronically difficult, infrequent, or incomplete defecation. Prevalence in people over the age of 65 is up to 50%. Laxatives to correct constipation are used by 50% to 75% of the residents of long-term care facilities. Constipation can be caused by certain medications and disorders, low-fiber diets, sedentary lifestyle or impaired mobility, tumors, or abdominal aortic aneurysm. Patients will complain of difficulty or inability to defecate. Constipation can lead to bowel obstruction, which may present with vomiting, diarrhea, and abdominal pain. Small bowel obstruction is a medical emergency.

Constipation Consideration

Medications such as loop diuretics, opioids, iron supplements, and calcium channel blockers are frequently associated with constipation in long-term care patients.

Fecal incontinence is a condition in which fecal matter leaks from the anus and bowel movements are not controlled. This can be caused by certain disorders, overuse of laxatives, constipation, muscle or nerve damage, diarrhea, or surgical complications.

Prehospital care is limited to supportive and empathetic care and includes transport to the ED or other appropriate facility. Chronic constipation or fecal incontinence not only can be embarrassing for the patient and family, but it also leads to a lower quality of life for the older adult patient due to associated medical complications.

Colorectal Cancer

Colorectal cancers are cancers of the colon and rectum. They are usually grouped together due to the similarities they share. Signs and symptoms include a persistent change in bowel habits, rectal bleeding, persistent abdominal pain, weakness or fatigue, and unexplained weight loss. Usually, the early stage of the disease is asymptomatic. Because of this, screening by colonoscopy is often done to detect the cancer while it is in the early stage and most treatable. Preparation for this screening can cause adverse effects such as fecal incontinence, abdominal pain, dizziness, nausea, and vomiting—a combination that may induce a call

Colorectal Cancer Concern

Colorectal cancer is the most frequent form of cancer in persons older than 75 years in the United States. Two-thirds of gastrointestinal cancers occur in persons over the age of 65.

to EMS. Increased risk of dehydration and electrolyte imbalances also occur with colonoscopy preparation.

Pancreatitis

Pancreatitis is an inflammatory disorder that results from premature activation of pancreatic enzymes, which causes the pancreas to begin digesting itself. Acute pancreatitis has a sudden onset and lasts for days, while chronic pancreatitis develops over years of repeated episodes of acute pancreatitis. There are many causes, including hypertriglyceridemia and medications such as amiodarone, carbamazepine, metronidazole, and quinolones (**FIGURE 6-3**).

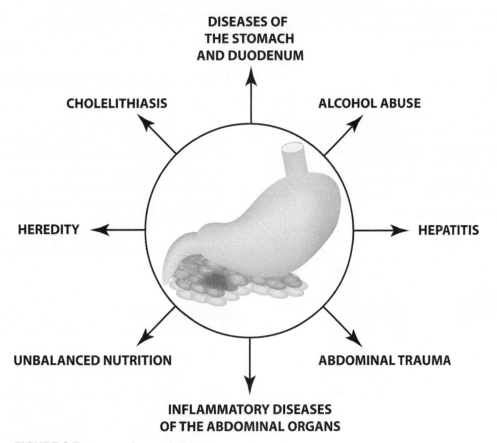

CAUSES OF PANCREATITIS

DISEASES OF
THE STOMACH
AND DUODENUM

CHOLELITHIASIS

ALCOHOL ABUSE

HEREDITY

HEPATITIS

UNBALANCED NUTRITION

ABDOMINAL TRAUMA

INFLAMMATORY DISEASES
OF THE ABDOMINAL ORGANS

FIGURE 6-3 Causes of pancreatitis.
© Timonina/Shutterstock

Acute signs and symptoms can include upper abdominal pain and tenderness, low-grade fever, tachycardia, and nausea and vomiting. Pancreatic bleeding can also cause the patient to present with **Cullen sign** or **Grey Turner sign**.

Prehospital treatment may include intravenous fluid administration, pain relief, and antiemetics.

Gallbladder Disease/Gallstones

Gallbladder disease has a high occurrence and high morbidity in the geriatric population, in part because the prevalence of gallstones is much higher in this group (**FIGURE 6-4**). Sharp right upper quadrant pain that often radiates to the back or right shoulder is the classic symptom associated with this disorder. Increased pain after eating fatty food is another common symptom of this disease. EMS practitioners should be concerned if a patient presents with right upper quadrant pain, fever, and possibly jaundice. This could be an indication of **cholangitis**, an infection in the gallbladder or entire biliary system, putting the patient at risk for sepsis and shock.

Severe Threats to Life

Older adults are at greater risk of developing complications from gallbladder disease, including death from surgical therapy.

Recall that geriatric patients often have atypical presentations. Proper prehospital care involves appropriate assessment to rule out other potential life-threatening causes of symptoms such as acute myocardial infarction (AMI). Once an AMI has been ruled out, prehospital care can involve pain management and antiemetic therapy. Follow your local protocols regarding emergent transport of these patients.

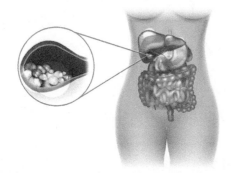

FIGURE 6-4 Gallstones.

Abdominal Aortic Aneurysm

Though technically not a GI disorder, abdominal aortic aneurysm (AAA) is a common cause of abdominal pain. As the body ages, atherosclerosis and hypertension both weaken the aortic walls while increasing the pressure against them. Weak points on the aorta are stretched and damaged, forming one or more bulges in the vessel wall called aneurysms (**FIGURE 6-5**). One such weak point is at the aorta located in the abdomen, inferior to the renal artery branches. Most AAAs do not leak, rupture, or dissect, and fewer than 50% of patients present with the classic signs and symptoms of abdominal or back pain, hypotension, and a pulsatile abdominal mass.

Assume the Worst-Case Scenario

Older adults complaining of abdominal or back pain should be assumed to have an AAA even if there is no pulsatile mass or hypotension.

Due to the potential for large amounts of blood to be lost through the damaged wall, patient survival will depend on the body's ability to form clots and a rapid transport to the closest facility with surgical capabilities, and possibly fluid resuscitation en route.

Herpes Zoster (Shingles)

As with AAA, herpes zoster, or shingles, is not a GI disorder. However, shingles can cause severe abdominal pain, especially if internal shingles develop. Shingles is a viral infection that causes a painful rash and is caused by reactivation of the herpes zoster virus (the same virus that causes chicken pox) on nerve roots. The current generation of older adults is very likely to have had chicken pox and so is at risk of developing shingles. Risk factors include cancer or immunosuppression, but even older adults in good health may develop shingles.

Even in Good Health, Get Your Vaccine

Risk and incidence increase with age. Every year, an estimated 1 million people in the United States get shingles, regardless of health status, and about one out of three people in the United States will develop shingles at some point. A shingles vaccine is recommended for all adults over age 50.

Normal   Abdominal Aortic Aneurysm

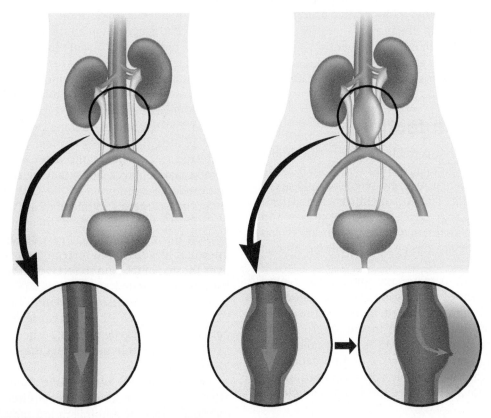

FIGURE 6-5 Abdominal aortic aneurysm.
© Alila Medical Media/Shutterstock

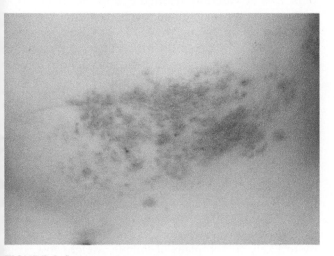

FIGURE 6-6 Herpes zoster (shingles).
© Franciscodiazpagador/iStock/Getty Images Plus/Getty Images

Signs and symptoms include a blistering rash with severe pain, itchiness, or tingling, which sometimes can precede the rash for days to weeks (**FIGURE 6-6**). Headaches, light sensitivity, and malaise may also be present before development of rash. The rash typically appears as a single strip of blisters that follows the affected nerve and wraps around either the right or left side of the torso. The blisters can also appear on the buttocks, legs, or face. Postherpetic neuralgia is the most common complication, with persistent pain in the area where the rash appeared. Additional complications include acute or chronic ophthalmic sequelae, bacterial superinfection of lesions, cranial and peripheral nerve palsies, and visceral involvement (e.g., pneumonia, hepatitis, acute retinal necrosis, etc.). The virus can spread with direct contact of the lesions, which can trigger varicella (chicken pox) rather than shingles in the exposed person.

Renal and Genitourinary Disorders

Urinary Retention and Incontinence

Twenty percent of residents in long-term care facilities report they have urinary incontinence. This tends to be more common in women and is thought to be underreported. Urinary retention is another common complaint in the geriatric population. Causes can be related to diabetic neuropathy, postoperative procedures, infection, immobility, pain, medications, or prostate issues. Chronic conditions like urinary retention and urinary incontinence lead to a lower quality of life for the older adult patient. Prehospital management involves supportive and empathetic care.

Urinary Tract Infection

Older adults are more susceptible to urinary tract infections (UTIs) due to an impaired immune system; weak bladder muscles, leading to urine retention and accumulation of bacteria; diabetes mellitus; an enlarged prostate; use of a urinary catheter; kidney stones; and urinary or fecal incontinence. If untreated, UTIs can lead to kidney damage, kidney failure, altered mental status, and sepsis.

Though older adults may have some of the typical signs and symptoms of a UTI, they often present atypically with confusion or altered mental status, falls, anorexia, and even sepsis. Due to the severe nature of these atypical symptoms, EMS is often called. Focus of prehospital care is to provide symptomatic care. Hospital-based care will include administration of antibiotics and removal of infected indwelling catheters.

The Usual Suspect

Always suspect a UTI, regardless of presentation.

Chronic Kidney Disease

Loss of renal function is associated with chronic kidney disease. Maintaining an awareness of complications associated with this disorder and how it is managed is essential for appropriate patient care. Clinical features of chronic kidney disease include edema, nausea and vomiting, dyspnea, chest discomfort, dysrhythmias, altered level of consciousness, and changes in urinary habits. Missing only a single dialysis treatment means the patient will have excess fluid and waste products in their bloodstream. This will put them at risk for fluid overload, presenting as dyspnea and pulmonary edema, as

From Function to Failure

Dialysis or a transplant is needed when 80% of the nephrons have been damaged. Recall that 50% are damaged through the normal aging process.

well as hyperkalemia, which can cause life-threatening arrythmia.

The incidence of chronic kidney disease, which leads to end-stage renal failure, is rapidly increasing in patients older than 75 years in the United States and other developed countries. Chronic kidney disease is linked to atherosclerosis, which means care for the patient is often complicated by comorbidities such as chronic heart failure, acute coronary syndromes, and myocardial infarctions, among other common conditions related to aging. Peritoneal dialysis may be the preferred treatment for the older adult, as it has less hemodynamic effect, but it may be contraindicated by aging-related conditions of the GI tract or history of abdominal surgeries. While dialysis is effective, it risks complications to the patient's vascular condition, hypotension during treatment, heart disease exacerbation, intestinal bleeding, and increased risk of stroke. Those over the age of 65 tend to receive catheters rather than fistulas to facilitate hemodialysis.

Prehospital assessment should include a 12-lead ECG to rule out AMI as the cause of symptoms. The patient should also be continuously monitored for dysrhythmias due to hyperkalemia that is associated with kidney failure.

Prehospital care can include fluid administration, although extreme caution is required to avoid fluid overload. Diuretic administration may be provided to enhance any remaining kidney function and increased the vascular space through vasodilation. Analgesics must also be carefully selected due to the reduced excretion causing toxic blood levels. Fentanyl has been approved for use by the World Health Organization for these types of patients. Pharmaceutical correction of life-threatening hyperkalemia can also be provided by advanced EMS practitioners.

Endocrine Disorders
Diabetes Mellitus

Geriatric diabetic patients are less likely to present with the classic symptoms of hyperglycemia such as **polyuria** (excessive urination), **polydipsia** (excessive thirst), and **polyphagia** (excessive hunger). They are more likely to complain of fatigue, weight loss, cognitive impairment, and altered sleep patterns. Patients

Type 2 = 1/3

Almost one-third of the U.S. geriatric population has type 2 diabetes.

over the age of 75 are twice as likely to go to the hospital due to hypoglycemia than are younger patients with diabetes.

Treatment of a geriatric patient with suspected or known diabetes is similar to that of younger patients. When suspecting a diabetic condition, assessment must include **glucometry**. Treatment of hypoglycemia involves rapid correction by the administration of glucose orally or dextrose intravenously. Hyperglycemic patients may require a fluid bolus if dehydrated. A fluid bolus of normal saline (500 ml/hr) can be considered for patients with severe hyperglycemia. Ensure renal and cardiac functions are reviewed prior to administering fluid. Watch closely for signs of fluid overload, which include edema, shortness of breath, hypertension, chest pain, abdominal cramps, and abdominal bloating.

Admission to an intensive care setting is usually required due to the need for IV insulin infusions and close monitoring during correction of severe metabolic disturbances.

Thyroid Disorders

The thyroid gland secretes the hormones tetraiodothyronine (T4) and triiodothyronine (T3). These hormones regulate body systems to maintain homeostasis. For example, the thyroid affects the resting heart rate and cardiac contractility, and therefore cardiac output. It also adjusts the breathing rate in response to hypoxia and hypercapnia. Body weight and energy are controlled through carbohydrate metabolism, lipid metabolism, GI motility, and renal water clearance.

Although thyroid disorders are twice as common in older adults, comorbidities and polypharmacy can mask symptoms and make identification difficult.

Hypothyroidism

Hypothyroidism is the most common thyroid disorder and involves a lack of hormone secretion. This condition can lead to constipation, weight gain, heat intolerance, anemia, and arrythmia. The most common complaints are fatigue and weakness. Hypothyroidism also may lead to edema, **angioedema** (puffy face), dry skin, **macroglossia** (large tongue), coarse hair, and hair loss (**FIGURE 6-7**). Medical treatment is hormone replacement and monitoring cardiac and nervous system functions. Long-term treatment includes hormone replacement.

Hyperthyroidism

Hyperthyroidism involves excessive hormone secretion, which can cause tachycardia, dyspnea, muscle weakness, angina, HF, and AMI (**FIGURE 6-8**). Other symptoms can include loss of appetite and diarrhea.

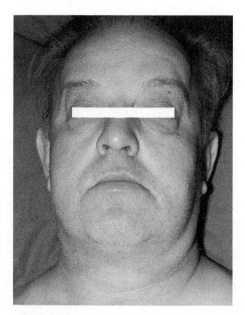

FIGURE 6-7 Localized accumulations of mucinous material in the neck of a hypothyroid patient.
Copyright © 2024 National Association of Emergency Medical Technicians (NAEMT).

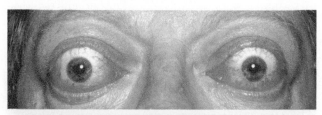
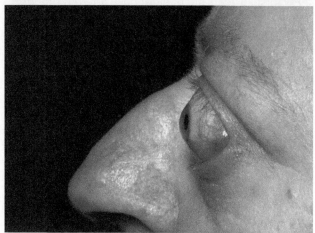

FIGURE 6-8 Note the bulging eyes characteristic of hyperthyroidism in these patients.
© Science Photo Library/Science Source; © SPL/Science Source

Medical treatment includes monitoring of cardiac function and administration of beta-adrenergic blockers for cardiac rhythm control, radioactive iodine to shrink the glands, antithyroid medications, or surgery to remove the glands. Similar to patients with hypothyroidism, prehospital care involves cardiac monitoring.

Thermoregulation Disorders

Hypothermia

Hypothermia is a reduction in the body's core temperature to < 95.0°F (< 35.0°C). Older adults are at a much higher risk of hypothermia due to their bodies' diminished ability to respond to changes in ambient temperature and maintain a normal temperature. For example, less insulation (less subcutaneous fat, less hair, thinner skin) reduces the ability of older adults to retain heat, and less muscle mass means they cannot shiver enough to help keep their body temperature up. Release of catecholamines, a heat source in the body, is also diminished due to the steady decline in metabolism.

Chronic medical conditions and certain medications also impact the older person's ability to cope with colder environments. For example, diabetic patients are six times more likely to suffer from hypothermia, in part due to vascular disease that alters thermoregulatory mechanisms. Additionally, people with mobility problems may not be able to seek shelter from the cold, and patients with dementia may not know how to make themselves warmer when they are cold.

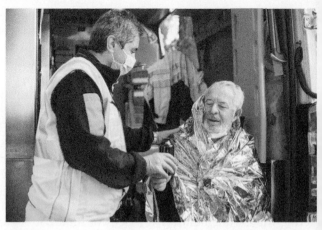

FIGURE 6-9 Always keep patients covered and warm, as older adults are at higher risk of developing hypothermia.
© loreanto/Shutterstock

Turn Up the Heat

Persons 75 years old or older have an even higher risk of death from hypothermia than other age groups and can become hypothermic indoors, even in mildly cool buildings with temperatures from 60° to 65° F (16° to 18° C).

Signs and symptoms vary and are often atypical. Patients may present with confusion, weakness, tachycardia (early sign), hypertension (early sign), lower core body temperature, and shivering occasionally (however, this sign may not be present). Treatment includes warming the patient, stabilization of airway, breathing, and circulation and removal from the cold environment (if applicable). Use caution when preparing the patient for transport to minimize the chance of triggering abnormal heart rhythms. Be sure to keep patients covered and warm at all times (**FIGURE 6-9**). Follow local protocols for resuscitation of hypothermic patients.

Hyperthermia

Hyperthermia occurs when the body is unable to get rid of heat buildup, often as a result of hot and humid conditions. Older adults' thermoregulation is negatively impacted by reduced functioning of sweat glands and decreased ability to cool off through perspiration. There are three major types of heat illness resulting from hyperthermia: heat cramps, heat exhaustion, and heatstroke. **Heatstroke** is the most severe form of heat illness, and is considered a profound emergency.

Too Hot to Handle

People over the age of 50 years account for 80% of all deaths from heatstroke, and these emergencies are 12 to 13 times more common in people 65 years and older. The number of deaths rises exponentially in those over age 65 years.

Patients with hyperthermia typically present with confusion, irritability, and combativeness. The pulse rate of older patients with heatstroke is usually very slow and thready, and the patient usually presents with hypovolemia. Treatment of older adults with hyperthermia is the same as for younger patients.

Electrolyte Disturbances

Older adults can maintain water and electrolyte balance when healthy, but maintaining water and electrolyte balance is more challenging than for younger patients during an illness, a decline in cognitive ability, or when exposed to extreme temperatures. Medications can also cause an imbalance to occur. For these reasons, electrolyte disturbances are common in older adults with preexisting medical conditions.

Dehydration

Though dehydration is not generally the main reason EMS is called for an older patient, you should always evaluate for it and administer treatment or transport in order to prevent worsening of the underlying cause and potential damage to other critical body systems.

Signs to look for include dry mucous membranes, flat neck veins, increased heart rate or low blood pressure, absence of urine output, or a weight that is significantly less than the patient's usual weight. Evaluation of skin turgor ("tenting") is very unreliable in older patients and should not be relied upon for evaluation.

Continuously monitor the patient's ECG. Abnormal vital signs must be treated as soon as possible. If the patient has an altered mental status and low blood pressure, IV fluids are required until the patient is stabilized. Evaluate glucose level and, if low, administer dextrose 50% according to your local protocol.

Early transport is urgent if your level of certification does not allow you to provide IV therapy. If you are certified to administer IV fluids, watch for fluid overload, which can damage other body systems. At times, establishing intravenous access can be difficult in an older person, whose veins tend to roll and may be collapsed because of low blood volume.

When preparing the patient for transport, pay close attention to the patient's skin condition. When dehydrated, the skin may be very thin and susceptible to tears and pressure ulcers.

Hyponatremia

Hyponatremia, a common electrolyte abnormality found in geriatric patients, is defined by a serum sodium concentration below 135 mEq/l. An older person is prone to this disorder due to water retention caused by renal deterioration, administration of medications that increase excretion of sodium; and, rarely, from disorders associated with hyponatremia, such as inappropriate antidiuretic hormone secretion.

Critical Thinking Question

How does renal impairment cause hyponatremia?

Signs and symptoms will vary depending on the rate and degree of change in sodium concentration. Patients can present with weakness, lethargy, hallucinations, agitation, seizures, abdominal cramps, headaches, and altered mental status. Severe electrolyte disturbances can be fatal if not treated promptly. There are different states of hyponatremia, including:

- **Hypervolemia**, which occurs when excess water is retained in relation to the amount of sodium.
- **Hypovolemia**, which is a loss of water and sodium where more sodium is lost in relation to water.
- **Euvolemic hyponatremia**, which occurs when serum osmolarity is low despite the presence of concentrated urine.

Prehospital care is limited to supportive care and transport. Fluids should be administered cautiously, as aggressive hydration without knowing the serum sodium level can cause neurologic damage. Hospital-based treatment depends on the cause of the imbalance and can include sodium replacement, discontinuation of certain medications, and fluid level monitoring with correction as needed.

Hyperkalemia

Potassium is the most prevalent intracellular cation and helps regulate chemical reactions and heart function. Hyperkalemia is common in older adults and occurs when a higher-than-normal concentration of potassium (> 5.5 mEql/l) is detected in the bloodstream. This imbalance can result from ingestion of potassium supplements, renal failure, following blood transfusion, acidosis, sepsis, certain medication use, or with Addison's disease. Medications that interfere with the excretion of potassium include potassium-sparing diuretics, angiotensin-converting enzyme inhibitors, renin inhibitors, angiotensin receptor blockers, heparin, and NSAIDs.

Signs and symptoms typically involve cardiac and neurologic dysfunction. These can include weakness, cramps, **tetany**, paralysis, palpitations, and potentially lethal arrythmias. Classic ECG findings associated with hyperkalemia include peaked and symmetrical T waves, widened QRS complexes, prolonged PR interval, flattened or absent P wave, and a sine-wave appearance of the rhythm (**FIGURE 6-10**).

Since severely high concentrations of potassium have distinctive ECG patterns and these levels are potentially lethal, many EMS services provide the same initial treatment as is done in the hospital. The treatment focuses on stabilizing the cell membranes to decrease outflow of potassium into the bloodstream, shifting the potassium back into the cells; excretion of excess potassium; and decreasing cardiac irritability. Nebulized albuterol can decrease a serum potassium level by 0.5–1.5 mEq/l immediately. This is beneficial when there are concerns of fluid overload, such as in a patient with renal failure. These treatments may be administered in conjunction with cardiac resuscitation if required.

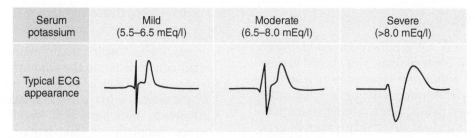

Serum potassium	Mild (5.5–6.5 mEq/l)	Moderate (6.5–8.0 mEq/l)	Severe (>8.0 mEq/l)
Typical ECG appearance			

FIGURE 6-10 ECG findings associated with hyperkalemia.

Copyright © 2024 National Association of Emergency Medical Technicians (NAEMT).

Sepsis

Sepsis is a systemic inflammatory immune response resulting from an infection. Sepsis can progress and cause organ failure, referred to as severe sepsis; hypotension; or septic shock. Septic shock most often occurs in the geriatric population.

A Deadly Threat

The World Health Organization reports that each year, sepsis affects 49 million people globally, leading to 11 million deaths. The Centers for Disease Control and Prevention reports at least 1.7 million American adults develop sepsis, and approximately 270,000 Americans die from sepsis every year.

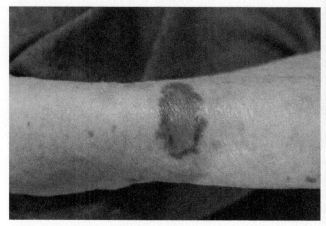

FIGURE 6-11 Classic finding of purpura rash associated with sepsis.

© A.UDOMRATSAK/Shutterstock

Sepsis can be caused by various infectious pathogens. Common infection sites include the skin and joints, lining of the central nervous system, lower respiratory tract, lining of the heart, the urinary tract, and **iatrogenic** infections caused by medical device placement. Sometimes there may be a clinical suspicion of infection, but the source is unknown.

The immune system response causes a cascading effect, first infiltrating the infected area with leukocytes to detect and destroy pathogens. Vasoactive substances are also secreted by the immune system, which leads to peripheral vasodilation and increased capillary permeability. This can lead to interstitial edema, hypovolemia, and hypoperfusion. Intravascular coagulation also occurs, which depletes the body's level of coagulation factor and worsens capillary leakage. This leads to the classic finding of a **purpura rash**, a nonblanching purplish discoloration of the skin (**FIGURE 6-11**).

Classic signs and symptoms of sepsis include fever and chills, localized pain at the infection site, nausea and vomiting, hematuria, purpura, coma, and seizures.

Atypical Presentation

Atypical signs and symptoms of sepsis in older adults include malaise, falls, dizziness, syncope, loss of balance, immobility, incontinence, paresis, difficulty speaking, and confusion.

However, sepsis will often present with atypical signs and symptoms in the geriatric population.

The systemic inflammatory response syndrome (SIRS) criteria include fever > 100.4°F (38°C) or hypothermia < 96.8°F (36°C), heart rate > 90 bpm, breathing rate > 20 rpm, and white blood cell count > 12,000/mm^3 or < 4,000/mm^3. While this assessment is appropriate for younger patients, the SIRS criteria are less able to identify severe infection in a geriatric patient, as the criteria may identify non-septic disorders such as asthma, dehydration, urinary tract infection, and sinus infection, because geriatric patients often have abnormal vital signs.

In severe sepsis, lactic acid is released into the bloodstream as a byproduct of anaerobic metabolism in hypoxic tissues. The increased lactic acid can be detected with a point-of-care lactate reading > 4 mmol/l. Tachypnea may also result from severe sepsis, which can lower $ETCO_2$ to < 25 mm Hg.

Rapid administration of antibiotics drastically improves the patient's prognosis. Many EMS agencies direct crews to alert the receiving hospital that sepsis is suspected. Some EMS agencies carry antibiotics to administer to these patients during transport.

A weight-based fluid resuscitation approach should be considered, as studies have shown that 20 to 30 ml/kg of crystalloid fluid administration within the first 1 to 2 hours demonstrated the lowest 28-day mortality rate.

In contrast, higher mortality was found in patients who received a larger fluid bolus. Care must be taken to closely monitor a geriatric patient during fluid administration, as too rapid an administration or administration of too much fluid can lead to heart failure or renal failure. Patients with existing heart or renal disease are at higher risk of becoming unstable with administration of a large amount of fluid.

Hospital administration of a vasopressor is indicated if the patient does not respond to the fluid resuscitation. A vasopressor is used to constrict peripheral blood vessels and reduce the vascular space as well as reduce fluid leakage from the capillaries. Norepinephrine is the vasopressor preferred for the treatment of septic shock.

CASE STUDY

You are dispatched to a senior living community residence for a 77-year-old female with altered mental status. It is a cool, fall evening. The air temperature is 50°F (10°C).

QUESTIONS

- What is your differential diagnosis?
  - Head trauma
  - Stroke
  - UTI
  - Hyperkalemia
  - Hypoglycemia
  - Renal failure
  - DKA
  - Toxicity
  - Dehydration

- How does the patient's age affect your assessment approach?
  - You should incorporate the GEMS diamond into your assessment.

As you arrive at the residence you are met by home health staff, who take you to the patient lying in bed in her room.

You determine the scene is safe and that you are wearing appropriate PPE. As you make your way through the residence you note it is well-kept and without significant obstacles. The temperature in the residence is warm.

You note that the patient wears glasses and dentures and appears to have proper nutrition and needed supplies in the residence. The patient appears lethargic and is slow to respond to verbal stimuli.

The staff member tells you that she is an aide for the senior living community and checks on the patient daily to assist with any needed ADLs. The aide also informs you the patient lives alone and manages her ADLs effectively. The patient receives meals from the senior living dining facility located in her community.

The staff aide tells you that the patient has not been feeling well and has complained of multiple muscle cramps in her legs with generalized weakness for 3 days now. The staff aide further reports that the patient is on dialysis and missed her last appointment. Today the patient presents with an altered mental status that is not normal for her, and she is expected to go to a dialysis appointment, but the staff aide is unable to arouse her.

QUESTION

- Do you have any concerns based on your findings so far?
  - Altered mental status is always a concern, especially in an older patient who is normally fully alert and oriented. The fact that the patient has missed a dialysis appointment should also raise concerns for electrolyte imbalances related to kidney failure.

You perform a primary survey that reveals the patient has a patent airway; is breathing fast and deeply with rales, or crackles, heard when auscultating both bases; and has a palpable radial pulse, which is regular and strong. You also note that she is lethargic, but responds to voice with eye opening and moaning and has equal and reactive pupils.

You perform the primary survey, which reveals the following:

- X–No bleeding found
- A–Patent
- B–Respirations are rapid and deep. Lung sounds reveal rales (crackles) in the bases bilaterally
- C–Radial pulse, regular and strong; skin is warm and dry.
- D–Lethargic, GCS 13 (E3, V4, M6); PERRL
- E–Pitting edema to both lower legs; AV fistula noted to the left arm. No other injuries noted on exposure.

QUESTIONS

- What is the cardinal presentation and the chief complaint?
  - Cardinal presentation: Altered mental status
  - Chief complaint: "Not feeling well," muscle cramps, weakness

- Is the AV fistula of concern?
  - You will need to remember to not use that arm when assessing blood pressure or for IV access.

- What could the rales indicate?
  - Rales indicate there may be fluid in the lungs, which could be a sign of pneumonia.

- Are any interventions required before assessment can continue?
  - No.

- Does this patient require immediate transport, or can you remain on scene and continue your assessment?
  - You elect to remain on scene and continue your assessment.

- Has your differential diagnosis changed?

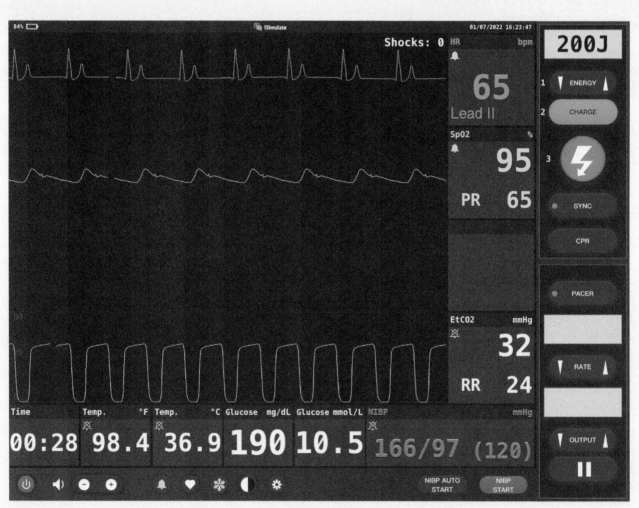

FIGURE 6-12

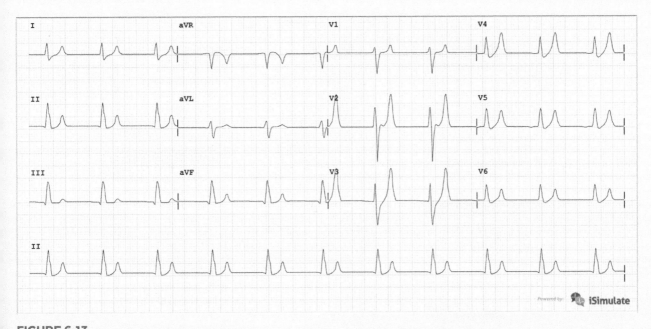

FIGURE 6-13

– Pneumonia may now be a concern; no evidence of head trauma.

- What further assessments would you like to perform?
  - You assess vital signs and take a detailed history and physical examination.

You further assess the patient by measuring blood pressure and attaching a cardiac monitor and oximeter. The results of these assessments are as follows:

- HR: 68
- BP: 170/98
- RR: 24
- Temp: 97.5°F (36.4°C) tympanic
- SpO$_2$: 95% on room air
- Glucometry: 190 mg/dl (10.5 mmol/l)

A 12-lead ECG reveals tall, peaked T waves, small P waves, and widened QRS complexes.

The patient is unable to communicate so the nurse tells you the patient has complained of generally feeling unwell for 3 days and complained of dizziness earlier today. The nurse says it seemed to have a gradual onset and is unable to provide further OPQRST information.

- O–Gradual
- P–None
- Q–Unable to assess
- R–Unable to assess
- S–Unable to assess
- T–3 days

The patient information sheets handed to you by the nurse indicate the patient has no allergies and is prescribed lisinopril, metformin, and hydrocodone-acetaminophen 5/500. Although the patient has been compliant with her medications, she missed her last dialysis appointment, meaning she has had no dialysis treatment for 4 days. The patient lives alone but has a home care aide visit daily to assist with activities of daily living (ADL) and receives meals from the community senior living dining facility.

You elicit the history of the cardinal presentation as best you can using the SAMPLER mnemonic.

- S–Altered mental status, muscle cramps, generalized weakness, bilateral rales
- A–None
- M–Lisinopril, metformin, hydrocodone-acetaminophen PRN for pain (has not taken today)
- P–HTN, diabetes type 2, chronic renal failure on dialysis 3 times/week.
- L–Ate soup and toast 2 days ago.
- E–Wasn't feeling well 3 days ago and missed last dialysis appointment 2 days ago.
- R–Age, renal failure, altered LOC

Prior to placing the patient on your stretcher, you conduct a head-to-toe physical exam (**FIGURE 6-14**), which is unremarkable except for an S3 gallop heart sound and the edema (**FIGURE 6-15**) and lung sounds noted in the primary survey.

Detailed Physical Exam

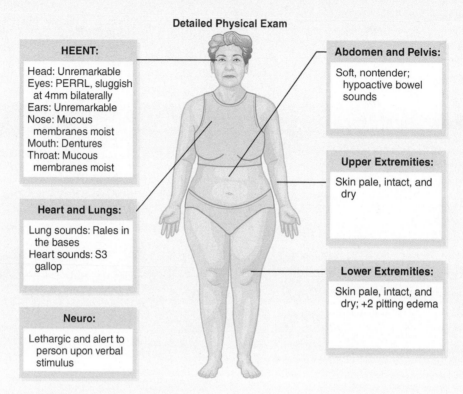

HEENT:

Head: Unremarkable
Eyes: PERRL, sluggish
  at 4mm bilaterally
Ears: Unremarkable
Nose: Mucous
  membranes moist
Mouth: Dentures
Throat: Mucous
  membranes moist

Abdomen and Pelvis:

Soft, nontender;
  hypoactive bowel
  sounds

Upper Extremities:

Skin pale, intact, and
  dry

Heart and Lungs:

Lung sounds: Rales in
  the bases
Heart sounds: S3
  gallop

Lower Extremities:

Skin pale, intact, and
  dry; +2 pitting edema

Neuro:

Lethargic and alert to
  person upon verbal
  stimulus

FIGURE 6-14 Physical assessment.
Copyright © 2024 National Association of Emergency Medical Technicians (NAEMT).

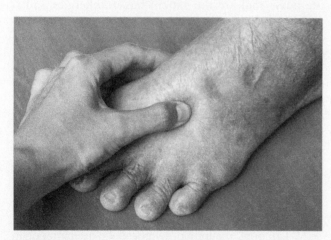

FIGURE 6-15 Pitting edema on the foot.
© Zay Nyi Nyi/Shutterstock

Prehospital Treatment

- BLS
  - Position of comfort
  - Oxygen
  - Consider albuterol breathing treatment
  - Glucose
  - Monitor vitals

- ALS
  - BLS care
  - IV therapy
  - Fluid TKVO

- Critical care
  - BLS/ALS care
  - Calcium chloride
  - Sodium bicarbonate

GEMS DIAMOND REVIEW

How was the GEMS Diamond information applied in this case?

 Geriatric Assessment: A 77-year-old female with consistent age-related changes.

 Environmental Assessment: The residence is well-kept with easy access. The temperature in the home is warm. No significant obstacles noted. No odors noted. The patient appears to have appropriate food, and needed supplies, and she also wears dentures and wears glasses.

Medical Assessment: The home health aide details several medical conditions, such as hypertension, type 2 diabetes, and chronic renal failure. The patient appears to be compliant with her medications.

Social Assessment: The patient lives alone; her husband died 3 years prior. She can accomplish most ADLs by herself, and a home health aide assists as needed. The patient receives her meals from the senior living dining facility located in her community.

QUESTIONS

- Where should this patient be transported?
  - This patient should be transported to the closest facility with dialysis capabilities.
- What other assessments are likely to be performed in the hospital?
  - A second ECG to compare with the first, along with blood and urine analysis.

- What is your goal for prehospital treatment?
  - ECG suggests hyperkalemia; if permitted by medical direction, medications to lower potassium levels (albuterol, calcium gluconate, sodium bicarbonate, dextrose, or insulin) could be administered. The ECG should be continuously monitored en route.

The patient is transported on a stretcher in a position of comfort to the closest facility with dialysis capabilities.

At the hospital, a second 12-lead ECG is performed and compared to the first, a Foley catheter inserted, and samples of blood and urine are collected for analysis. Diuretics are administered to eliminate excess potassium and fluids. Arrangements are made for hemodialysis should the pharmacologic therapies fail to lower and eliminate potassium sufficiently.

The patient is admitted to the hospital for treatment of hyperkalemia. She receives care to correct the hyperkalemia, counseling on the importance of dialysis treatments, and her social supports are assessed.

CASE STUDY WRAP-UP

Patients with renal failure who miss a single dialysis treatment are at risk for dangerous levels of potassium in the bloodstream as well as fluid overload. High levels of potassium in the blood destabilize the cardiac cell's ability to depolarize and repolarize normally. This can lead to life-threatening arrythmias that are refractory to treatment until potassium levels are lowered. Dialysis is the preferred method to correct hyperkalemia, so transport to a facility with dialysis capabilities is required.

CHAPTER WRAP-UP

Abdominal pain is one of the leading causes for geriatric ED visits. As with younger patients, the complexity of the abdominal anatomy and physiology combined with vague and variable clinical features make the assessment of abdominal discomfort challenging without advanced diagnostics. Prehospital care is therefore limited to providing supportive care and transport to the most appropriate facility.

Pharmacokinetics plays an important role in the management of abdominal disorders in geriatric patients. Decreased metabolism in the liver and decreased elimination of drug metabolites through the kidneys requires adjustment to drug dosing to avoid unintended toxic effects.

Early identification of potential GI, GU, metabolic, and electrolyte disorders can reduce mortality and improve recovery times. Early identification of sepsis is important, as septic shock most often occurs in the geriatric population.

REFERENCES

Isalimy N, Madi L. Efficacy and safety of laxatives for chronic constipation in long-term care settings: a systematic review. *J Clin Pharm Ther.* 2018;43(5):595–605.

Boyle P, Leon M. Epidemiology of colorectal cancer. *Br Med Bull.* 2002;64:1–25.

Buemi M, Lacquaniti A, Bolignano D, et al. Dialysis and the elderly: an underestimated problem. *Kidney Blood Press Res.* 2008;31(5):330–336.

Dumic I, Nordin T, Jecmenica M, Stojkovic Lalosevic M, Milosavljevic T, Milovanovic T. Gastrointestinal tract disorders in older age. *Can J Gastroenterol Hepatol*. 2019;2019:1–19. doi:10.1155/2019/6757524

Enzinger PC, Mayer RJ. Gastrointestinal cancer in older patients. *Semin Oncol*. 2004;31(2):206–219. doi:10.1053/j.seminoncol.2003.12.031

Filippatos TD, Makri A, Elisaf MS, Liamis G. Hyponatremia in the elderly: challenges and solutions. *Clin Interv Aging*. 2017;12:1957–1965.

Grundy SM. Metabolic syndrome update. *Trends Cardiovasc Med*. 2016;26(4):364–373.

Lyon C, Clark D. Diagnosis of acute abdominal pain in older patients. *Am Fam Physician*. 2006;74(9):1537–1544.

Malik RD, Cohn JA, Bales GT. Urinary retention in elderly women: diagnosis & management. *Curr Urol Rep*. 2014;15(11):454. doi:10.1007/s11934-014-0454-x

National Association of Emergency Medical Technicians. *AMLS: Advanced Medical Life Support: An Assessment-Based Approach*. 3rd ed. Burlington, MA: Jones & Bartlett Learning; 2021.

National Heart, Lung, and Blood Institute. What is metabolic syndrome? https://www.nhlbi.nih.gov/health-topics/metabolic-syndrome. Published date unknown. Accessed April 27, 2021.

Ng K, Lee C. Updated treatment options in the management of hyperkalemia. *US Pharm*. 2017;42(2):HS15–HS18. https://www.uspharmacist.com/article/updated-treatment-options-in-the-management-of-hyperkalemia. Published February 16, 2017. Accessed on May 15, 2022.

Norton P, Brubaker L. Urinary incontinence in women. *Lancet*. 2006 Jan; 367(9504):57–67.

Pilotto A, Franceschi M, Maggi S, Addante F, Sancarlo D. Optimal management of peptic ulcer disease in the elderly. *Drugs Aging*. 2010;27(7):545–558. doi:10.2165/11537380-000000000-00000

Pitchumoni CS, Dharmarajan TS. Abdominal pain. *Geriatric Gastroenterology*. Published online December 3, 2019:1–10. doi:10.1007/978-3-319-90761-1_43-1

Reid JR, Wheeler SF. Hyperthyroidism: diagnosis and treatment. *Am Fam Physician*. 2005 August;72(4):623–630.

Saad MAN, Cardoso GP, Martins WA, Velarde LGC, Cruz Filho RA. Prevalence of metabolic syndrome in elderly and agreement among four diagnostic criteria. *Arq Bras Cardiol*. Published online 2014. doi:10.5935/abc.20140013

Schlanger LE, Bailey JL, Sands JM. Electrolytes in the aging. *Adv Chronic Kidney Dis*. 2010;17(4):308–319. doi:10.1053/j.ackd.2010.03.008

Shaheen N, National Institute of Diabetes and Digestive and Kidney Diseases. Acid reflux (GER and GERD) in adults. https://www.niddk.nih.gov/health-information/digestive-diseases/acid-reflux-ger-gerd-adults. No date provided. Accessed on May 13, 2022.

Shami A. Heart failure causing postprandial abdominal pain in a young patient. *J Hosp Med*. 2017 May;12(2).

Spangler R, Van Pham T, Khoujah D, Martinez JP. Abdominal emergencies in the geriatric patient. *Int J Emerg Med*. 2014;7(1):43. doi:10.1186/s12245-014-0043-2

Vogel SL. Urinary incontinence in the elderly. *Ochsner J*. 2001;3(4):214–218. https://www.ncbi.nlm.nih.gov/pmc/articles/PMC3116748/. Published October 2001. Accessed April 27, 2021.

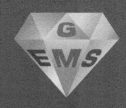

CHAPTER 7

Neurologic Emergencies

LESSON OBJECTIVES

- Describe the neurologic assessment of the older patient.
- Demonstrate the use of the GEMS Diamond in the neurologic assessment of the older patient.
- Discuss causes of altered mental status in the older patient.

- Review common neurologic emergencies in geriatric patients.
- Differentiate delirium from dementia.

Introduction

Issues related to nervous system dysfunction are common in older adults, due to aging nervous system cells that are not replaced during a lifetime. With time, the ability to create, repair, and replace synapses decreases, and dysfunction occurs. The rate of deterioration varies by individual, previous injury, amount of neural reserve, and whether nervous system disease is present.

A Disabling Problem

Older adults with neurologic dysfunction are potentially at higher risk for and suffer more falls than their counterparts without neurologic disease and dysfunction, increasing their risk for life-threatening injuries.

Brain Anatomy and Physiology Changes Due to Aging

Recall from Chapter 1: Changes with Age that the brain shrinks with age due to a selective loss of up to 50% of neurons and shrinkage of the remaining neurons. This shrinkage, or atrophy, can result in an estimated 25% loss of deep sleep and up to 55% loss of short-term memory. Loss of up to 20% of frontal lobe synapses can affect cognitive functions. Extra space within the skull means that elevating intracranial pressure due to brain swelling, intracranial hemorrhage, or intracranial mass may remain asymptomatic for a longer period of time before clinical signs and symptoms become apparent.

Critical Thinking Question

The brain shrinks 20% by age 80, but the skull does not. What happens to the extra space within the skull?

Brain Vasculature

Large internal carotid arteries feed 80% of the cerebrum. Vertebral arteries join the basilar artery inside the skull. Blockage of one of these arteries can cause reduced blood flow to the brain and result in a stroke.

The circle of Willis combines the posterior and anterior blood supplies to equalize blood pressure throughout the brain. It also helps ensure blood flow by providing an alternate route for blood flow to the brain if an artery becomes occluded.

Altered Mental Status

Altered mental status (AMS) is not a specific diagnosis. It describes a group of signs and symptoms of conditions such as cognitive disorders, attention disorders, arousal disorders, and decreased level of consciousness. The AEIOU-TIPS mnemonic was created to remind health care practitioners of the various causes of AMS (**TABLE 7-1**).

Mortality Factors

According to the World Health Organization, neurologic disorders are responsible for 12% of deaths globally.

In some ways, assessing an older patient for altered mental status is similar to assessing patients in other age groups. You should ask about current or recurring symptoms, such as headache or neck stiffness; and signs, such as body rash. You also need to ask about recent events, such as travel, trauma, infection, and possible exposure to toxins.

However, geriatric assessment is more challenging than assessing younger ages due to complicating conditions such as remote trauma or preexisting medical conditions. Before assessing the older patient, determine the patient's baseline mental status to which current and future findings can be compared. Comorbidities and medications often affect mentation, so medical history, current prescriptions, and recent changes to prescriptions must also be investigated.

Two other useful mnemonics used to remind EMS practitioners of potential pathologic causes of altered mental status are 4S and SNOT (**TABLES 7-2** and **7-3**).

Neurologic Disorders

Most neurologic disorders are not specific to the geriatric population; however, the prevalence of these disorders increases with age due to age-related deterioration and higher incidence of comorbidities.

Stroke

Stroke, also referred to as cerebrovascular accident, is a neurologic injury with a cardiovascular cause. The term cerebrovascular accident is not preferred by neurologists, as strokes are not accidents. A stroke occurs when blood flow to an area of the brain is disrupted

TABLE 7-1 AEIOU TIPS	
Mnemonic Component	AMS Cause
A	Alcohol, acidosis, ammonia, arrythmia
E	Electrolytes, endocrine, epilepsy, embolism
I	Infection or inflammation
O	Overdose, oxygen, opiates
U	Uremia
T	Temperature, trauma, thiamine
I	Insulin (hypo/hyperglycemia)
P	Psychiatric, poisoning
S	Stroke, seizure, syncope, space-occupying lesions, shunt malfunction, subarachnoid hemorrhage

TABLE 7-2 4S		
S	Sugar—check blood glucose levels	
S	Stroke—perform a stroke exam	
S	Seizure—is the patient currently having, or recently had, a seizure?	
S	Sepsis—look for signs of sepsis	

TABLE 7-3 SNOT	
S	Sugar, stroke, seizure, sepsis
N	Narcosis (CO_2, opiates)
O	Oxygen
T	Trauma, toxins, temperature

Note: This list is not comprehensive of all possible causes of altered mental status.

ISCHEMIC AND HEMORRHAGIC STROKE

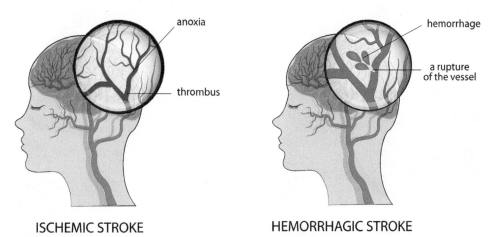

FIGURE 7-1 Ischemic versus hemorrhagic stroke.
© Artemida-psy/Shutterstock

due to blood clot becoming trapped in a cerebral artery, resulting in an ischemic stroke, or a cerebral artery rupturing and compressing surrounding cells, resulting in a hemorrhagic stroke (**FIGURE 7-1**). Most hemorrhagic strokes are intracerebral in that they occur within the brain tissue. Hemorrhagic strokes less frequently occur in the subarachnoid space.

Most Strokes Are Ischemic

Eighty-seven percent of strokes are ischemic.

Signs and symptoms of stroke include sudden onset of numbness, weakness, or paralysis to one side of the body, slurred speech, confusion, vision difficulty in one or both eyes, dizziness, ataxia, and severe headache with no apparent cause.

The more common ischemic strokes can be effectively reversed with thrombolytic therapy, which dissolves the offending clot and restores circulation if it is administered within 4.5 hours of symptom onset. Thrombolytic therapy administered to a patient experiencing an ischemic stroke can be lifesaving, but its administration to a hemorrhagic stroke patient would be catastrophic. Distinguishing an ischemic stroke from a hemorrhagic stroke by physical assessment alone is difficult; a patient must have a computed tomography (CT) scan to confirm the type of stroke before thrombolytics can be given. Larger blocked cerebral arteries can receive endovascular interventions, which are deemed safer than thrombolytics.

The key prehospital intervention for this type of patient is to identify suspected stroke symptoms, confirm the timing of the symptom onset, and provide rapid transport to the most appropriate facility if thrombolytics can be given in less than 4.5 hours.

Transient Ischemic Attack

A transient ischemic attack (TIA), also called a ministroke, involves a transient disruption of cerebral blood flow. A TIA will present exactly like a stroke but will resolve within 24 hours (**FIGURE 7-2**). A TIA is a critical risk factor for an impending stroke.

Warning: Stroke Ahead

Up to 15% of those who have a TIA will have a stroke within 3 months and 12% will die within 12 months.

Stroke Assessment

Given the importance of stroke identification in the prehospital setting, many stroke assessment tools have been developed to provide efficient and accurate identification. Three of these are RACE, CPSS, and BEFAST.

The **Rapid Arterial oCculsion Exam (RACE)** is used in the prehospital setting to identify stroke severity and strokes likely involving a large artery occlusion. Identification of this type of stroke allows transport to a facility with mechanical thrombectomy capability. The five items assessed are (1) facial palsy; (2) neurolinguistic dysfunction—specifically, aphasia or agnosia; (3) leg

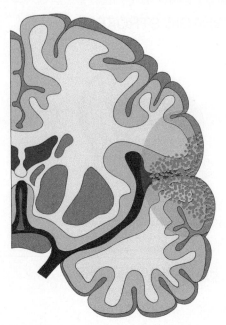
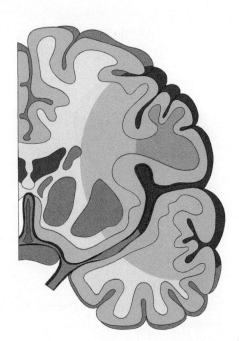

FIGURE 7-2 Transient ischemic attack (TIA).
© Double Rain/Shutterstock

motor function; (4) arm motor function; and (5) head/gaze deviation. Each item is scored on ability to fully perform a task, ability to partially perform a task, or inability to perform a task. The tool is scored out of 9 with a perfect score being 0. A score of 5 or higher indicates the likelihood of large vessel occlusion.

The **Cincinnati Prehospital Stroke Scale (CPSS)** tool is commonly used by prehospital practitioners. This assessment consists of testing for facial droop, arm drift, and abnormal speech. Eighty percent of stroke patients will exhibit one or more of these symptoms.

BEFAST is another mnemonic that can be used to identify stroke signs (AHORA [andar, hablar, ojos, rostro, ambos brazos] is the Spanish version) (**TABLE 7-4**). This tool can detect more than 95% of patients with ischemic stroke.

Stroke Treatment

There are four levels of stroke care available in most areas (**TABLE 7-5**).

Bell Palsy

Bell palsy is an unexplained episode of facial muscle weakness or paralysis that begins suddenly and worsens over 48 hours. Although it can occur at any age, it most commonly affects patients between 15 and 60 years old. It is thought to be an autoimmune disease attacking the nerves controlling facial movement

TABLE 7-4 BEFAST

BEFAST	
Balance	Sudden loss of balance, dizziness
Eyes	Vision loss or diplopia
Face	Facial droop or numbness, unequal smile
Arm	Weakness of one arm
Speech	Aphasia or dysarthria
Time	Time of symptom onset

Copyright © 2024 National Association of Emergency Medical Technicians (NAEMT).

Facial Droop: Bell Palsy or Stroke?

- A patient experiencing a stroke will be able to move their eyebrows normally despite having an unequal smile. Patients experiencing stroke also retain the ability to blink.
- A patient with Bell palsy will have asymmetrical movement and will not be able to raise the eyebrow on the drooping side of their face. Patients with Bell palsy are unable to blink (and therefore experience dry eyes).

TABLE 7-5 Levels of Stroke Care

Type of Hospital	Stroke Care Provided
1. Stroke-ready hospital	Rapid assessment including CT scan Ability to consult with neurologist Administration of thrombolytics Protocols for standardized care Typically transfers patients who receive thrombolysis
2. Primary stroke center	Rapid assessment including CT scan with advanced imaging Ability to consult with neurologist Administration of thrombolytics Protocols for standardized care May admit patients who receive thrombolysis
3. Thrombectomy-capable stroke center	Advanced imaging capabilities (CT, computed tomography angiography [CTA], magnetic resonance angiography [MRA]) Administration of thrombolytics Protocols for standardized care Admits patients who receive thrombolysis Dedicated vascular neurologist Can perform endovascular procedures
4. Comprehensive stroke center	Advanced imaging capabilities (CT, CTA, MRA) Administration of thrombolytics Protocols for standardized care Admits patients who receive thrombolysis Dedicated vascular neurologists and neurosurgeons Can perform endovascular procedures Dedicated neuro ICU beds Experience with managing stroke patients

(**FIGURE 7-3**). It may also be due to inflammation, compression, or swelling of cranial nerve VII, the facial cranial nerve. Bell palsy most often occurs in patients who have diabetes, influenza, upper respiratory illness, Guillain-Barré syndrome, multiple sclerosis, herpes simplex, or Lyme disease.

Seizures

A seizure is a transient occurrence of excessive or synchronous neuronal activity in the cerebral cortex that leads to a variable alteration in consciousness, muscle movement, incontinence, behavior change, subjective changes in perception (taste, smell), fears, and other symptoms (**FIGURE 7-4**). Seizures are classified as focal or generalized.

The prevalence and incidence of **epilepsy** and seizures increase correspondingly with increasing age. New-onset epilepsy in older adults typically has an underlying cause or precipitating disorder, including stroke, brain tumors, traumatic brain injury, and cerebrovascular diseases.

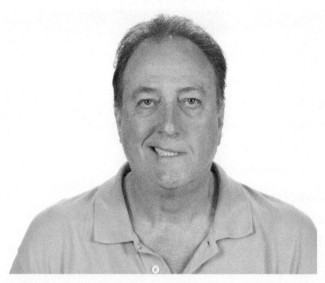

FIGURE 7-3 Facial paralysis and droop with inability to raise the eyebrow on the drooping side of face, indicative of Bell palsy.
© Steven Frame/Shutterstock

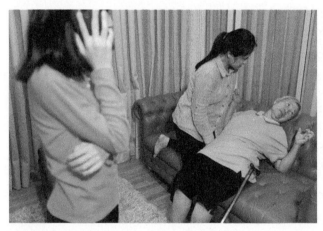

FIGURE 7-4 Older woman suffering a seizure.
© CGN089/Shutterstock

Seizure causes can include fever, infection, toxic drug ingestion or drug withdrawal, acute neurologic insult such as caused by a metabolic disorder, structural changes such as tumor formation, and congenital disorders. Epilepsy is diagnosed when a persistent abnormality in the brain causes recurrent seizures. Transient abnormalities such as hyponatremia or drug withdrawal are not considered to be epilepsy.

Unknown Origins

Approximately 70% of seizures have no known cause.

Focal Seizures

A focal seizure (previously called a partial seizure) involves a localized area of the brain. There are two subsets of focal seizures:

- Focal seizure with retained consciousness and awareness. Patients are usually awake and aware of seizure activity.
- Focal seizure without retained consciousness and awareness. Patients remain conscious during seizure activity but are unaware of their surroundings. Behaviors can range from quiet automatisms to aggressive and violent responses.

Prehospital management of focal seizures should include careful documentation, including talking with bystanders. The phrase "observe, contain, and don't restrain" has been used to remind practitioners that patients experiencing a focal seizure may have a violent reaction to physical touch or restraint.

Generalized Seizure

A generalized seizure involves both hemispheres of the brain and is associated with loss of consciousness. Generalized seizures are classified as follows:

- Absence (petit mal): staring spells often mistaken for daydreaming
- Atonic: sudden loss of muscle tone
- Tonic: flexion or extension of the head, trunk, or extremities
- Clonic: rhythmic motor jerking of the extremities or neck
- Tonic-clonic (grand mal): begin as tonic seizures and then become clonic, resolving when the patient becomes postictal

A secondary generalized seizure begins in one part of the brain and then spreads to both sides. This type of seizure will appear as a focal seizure followed by a generalized seizure.

Seizure Phases and Treatment

Depending on the type of seizure, up to three phases can occur.

1. The initial phase may be the preictal period in which the patient senses a hallucination or becomes aware that a seizure is about to occur.
2. The ictal phase occurs in all types of generalized seizure and is the period in which the seizure motor activity or behavior occurs.
3. The final phase may be the postictal period. In this period the seizure activity ceases and any alteration in consciousness gradually resolves.

Most seizure episodes resolve within 2 minutes and, although dramatic, are not life-threatening. Persistent seizure activity is defined as multiple ictal episodes without a return to normal level of consciousness between episodes. This condition is referred to as status epilepticus and it can be life-threatening.

For most seizures, the ictal phase has ended before EMS arrives. Therefore, prehospital care is often limited to supportive care and protection. Patients in the immediate postictal phase may not have returned to baseline mental status and EMS practitioners will need to rely on bystanders for a history of the event and precipitating factors. If the ictal phase is occurring on EMS arrival, protect the patient from self-harm during the seizure activity. Prehospital practitioners should assess whether the seizure episode is due to hypoglycemia or hypoxia and, if so, reverse either condition.

A detailed and objective description of seizure activity can be very helpful for physician and neurologist assessment. Due to its life-threatening nature, status epilepticus and any ictal phase persisting longer than 2 minutes are treated in the prehospital setting with the administration of a sedative. Hospital-based care involves sedation to calm ictal activity, identification of the cause, correction of the cause, and management of ictal activity with anticonvulsant or surgical therapy.

Neuropathy

More than 20 million people in the United States have some form of peripheral neuropathy. The exact number is difficult to determine as there is no definitive diagnostic test and the condition is often misdiagnosed due to the variety of possible symptoms.

Neuropathy is the result of damage to peripheral nerves due to trauma, infection, metabolic abnormalities such as those resulting from poor diabetic care, exposure to toxins, and vitamin deficiency. Peripheral nerve impulses can be disrupted by complete loss of signal, inappropriate signaling, and distortion of the messages being sent.

Symptoms can include weakness or pain in hands or feet that is described as stabbing, burning, or tingling. Symptoms can range from mild to disabling, but rarely are life-threatening.

Prehospital management is limited to providing pain relief and supportive care.

Parkinson Disease

More than 10 million people globally are living with Parkinson disease. Parkinson disease (PD) is a neurodegenerative disorder affecting mostly the dopaminergic neurons within the brain. The four classic signs are:

1. Tremors when at rest
2. Rigidity

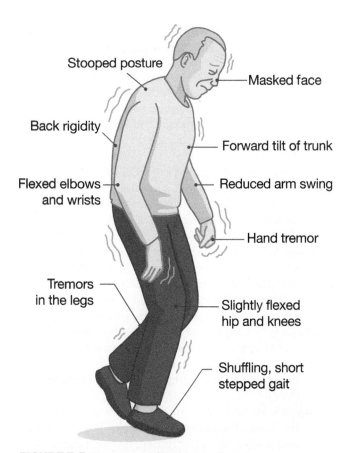

FIGURE 7-5 Symptoms of Parkinson disease.
© solar22/Shutterstock

3. Bradykinesia
4. Postural instability

There are five stages of PD, with symptoms increasing in each stage (**FIGURE 7-5**).

Patients with PD are susceptible to infections, as well as cardiovascular, cerebrovascular, and gastrointestinal disorders. EMS may be called to respond to patients with PD who have trauma from a fall.

Higher Age = Higher Incidence

The incidence of PD increases with age, affecting 3% of those over the age of 80.

Delirium

Delirium is a temporary abnormal sensorium with causes such as ethyl alcohol and barbiturate intoxication or withdrawal, trauma, seizure, endocrine disorders, encephalitis, sleep deprivation, and medication effect. It usually has an abrupt onset, and symptoms

Five Stages of Parkinson Disease

Stage 1. The first stage involves mild symptoms that typically do not interfere with daily activities. Abnormal movement like bradykinesia (slowness of movement), tremor, and rigidity occurs on one side of the body.

Stage 2. Clinical features progress to both sides of the body in stage 2. Although the activities of daily living can still be performed, difficulty ambulating and poor posture may be observed.

Stage 3. The third stage involves loss of balance and slow movements. The patient can still complete most activities of daily living but will have difficulty eating and dressing. Falls become more common in this stage.

Stage 4. The signs and symptoms become more severe in stage 4. The patient's movement becomes limited, so assistance is required to ambulate and perform activities of daily living.

Stage 5. Stage 5 is the most debilitating stage. At this stage, the patient is unable to stand or walk and is likely to be bedridden. Hallucinations and delusions may be experienced in this final stage.

TABLE 7-6 Delirium versus Dementia

Delirium	Dementia
Abrupt onset	Gradual onset
Temporary; symptoms can fluctuate over 24 hours	Permanent or progressive
Disorganized thinking and attention	Impaired recent memory and intellect
	Regression
Decreased consciousness	Normal consciousness
Impaired orientation	Impaired orientation
Hallucinations (visual, auditory)	No hallucinations
Delusions	No delusions
Increased motor movements	Movement is typically normal
Kinetic tremors	

Copyright © 2024 National Association of Emergency Medical Technicians (NAEMT).

can fluctuate over 24 hours. Symptoms include disorganized thinking, decreased consciousness, impaired orientation, visual and auditory hallucinations, disordered attention, impaired language expression, delusions, increased motor movements, and kinetic tremors. Patients may experience a fluctuating level of awareness over brief periods, and speech may be incoherent, tense, or rambling. Prehospital practitioners may note alterations in vital signs due to the underlying cause (e.g., infection, dehydration, intoxication). Patients must be fully evaluated and the root cause addressed. Patients who are in an acute state may require physical restraint and/or chemical sedation with a benzodiazepine or antipsychotic agent. Patients should be further assessed and managed in the ED.

Dementia

Dementia involves a chronic and irreversible loss of cognitive functioning to an extent that interferes with the capability of the person to perform daily activities. Onset of symptoms is gradual and progressive, involving impaired short-term memory and intellect, judgment, and orientation. Unlike delirium, the patient remains alert and has no hallucinations or delusions. Major differences between delirium and dementia are identified in **TABLE 7-6**.

Alzheimer Disease

Alzheimer disease is the most common form of dementia in the United States.

Due to presenting with similar symptoms, dementia is often confused with traumatic brain injury. To assist with differential diagnosis, determine if there is any history or possible history of recent head trauma such as from falls or motor vehicle collisions. Prehospital treatment is supportive and may include reassuring the patient and asking simple questions.

Comprehensive Neurologic Exam

A patient who appears alert and oriented may not have a normal mental status. These patients can still have alteration of judgment and understanding that needs to be elicited by a thorough neurologic assessment. A comprehensive neurologic exam includes assessment of mental status, cranial nerves, motor function, sensory function, reflexes, and cerebellar function. Comprehensive neurologic exams are not routinely performed in the prehospital setting. Cranial nerves and reflex function are rarely assessed in the prehospital setting, so they are not included here.

Mental Status

This assessment tests for wakefulness, orientation, and cognition. Assessment consists of asking simple questions to determine the patient's orientation. In the prehospital setting, the mental status assessment is limited to assessing a Glasgow Coma Scale score plus recollection of events from the onset of symptoms to the arrival of EMS. This is often referred to as "alert and oriented × 4" or "A&O×4," with the four elements being person, place, time, and events.

Before assessing a geriatric patient, determine the patient's normal baseline status from the patient's family or caregiver. For instance, it may not be appropriate to ask what day of the week it is if the patient does not follow a weekly schedule. A better question might involve the current season or most recent holiday. If the patient is normally confused as to the date, then record the assessment as you find it with a note that this is normal for the patient. This indicates that the patient has an altered mental status that has not deteriorated from their baseline.

Motor Function

Motor function is evaluated by testing all extremities for bilateral equality and strength, noting movement abnormalities such as flaccidity, spasticity, rigidity, or clonus. Testing is accomplished by having the patient perform specific tasks. This assessment requires the patient to be alert and cooperative. The arm drift exam may be used to evaluate patients suspected of having a stroke (**FIGURE 7-6**). Patients are asked to close their eyes and extend their arms with palms up. Note any downward drift or drop or any inward rotation of either arm.

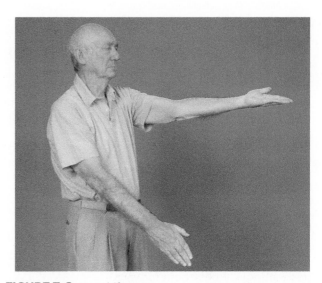

FIGURE 7-6 Arm drift test.

Sanders MJ: Mosby's paramedic textbook, revised reprint, ed 3, St. Louis, MO, 2007, Mosby

Sensory Function

The sensory function test evaluates the ability of the patient to sense touch, pain, and temperature stimulus on a dermatome. Touch is typically tested by touching the skin with a piece of tissue or cotton swab. Baseline function may be needed prior to assessment for patients with high likelihood of preexisting neuropathy, such as those with diabetes.

Cerebellar Function

This assessment involves evaluating the patient's balance and gait. This test is conducted by having the patient perform specific tasks that require intact cerebellar function. This test requires the patient to be alert and cooperative. Certain tasks will also require the patient to be ambulatory. Gait disturbance may be due to neurologic dysfunction, inner ear or spinal cord pathology, or muscle weakness. The patient, family member, or caregiver may report any of the following patient symptoms:

- Trouble coordinating movements
- Diplopia or irregular eye movements
- Feels weak or unstable when walking or standing

There may also be associated symptoms with incontinence, nausea, or visual changes. See **TABLE 7-7** for information about causes of ataxia.

Cerebellar function examination is not routinely performed prehospitally as the findings do not alter care or transport decisions.

TABLE 7-7 Causes of Ataxia

Gait Disturbance	Description	Differential Diagnosis
Broad-based gait	Person walks with an abnormally wide distance between the feet, which increases stability Patient may hesitate, freeze, lurch, or be unable to walk in a straight line	Acute alcohol intoxication Cerebellar atrophy caused by chronic alcohol abuse Diabetic peripheral neuropathy Stroke Ingestion of antiseizure medications such as phenytoin (Dilantin) Normal-pressure hydrocephalus Increased intracranial pressure
Propulsive (festinating) gait	Stooped, rigid posture, with the head and neck bent forward Shuffling gait Often accompanied by urinary incontinence	Advanced Parkinson disease Carbon monoxide poisoning Chronic exposure to manganese (in those who handle pesticides and in welders and miners) Ingestion of certain medications such as antipsychotics
Spastic gait	Characterized by stiffness and foot dragging Caused by long-term unilateral muscle contraction	Stroke Liver failure Spinal cord trauma or tumor Brain abscess or tumor Head trauma
Scissors gait	Crouching posture, with legs flexed at the hips and knees Knees and thighs brush together in a scissors-like movement when patient walks Patient takes short, slow, deliberate steps Patient may walk on toes or on balls of feet	Stroke Liver failure Spinal cord compression Thoracic or lumbar tumor Multiple sclerosis Cerebral palsy
Steppage gait	Characterized by foot drop; foot hangs down, causing toes to scuff the ground while walking	Guillain-Barré syndrome Lumbar disk herniation Peroneal nerve trauma

CASE STUDY

It is 1600 on a cold winter afternoon. You and your partner are staffing an emergency response ambulance and are dispatched to a house for an 81-year-old male with an altered mental status.

QUESTIONS

- What conditions are on your differential diagnosis list?
  - Altered level of consciousness can be from a range of causes. Some possibilities include:
    - AMI
    - Stroke
    - Infection
    - Toxins (i.e., narcotics, psychiatric meds)
    - Metabolic (diabetic, electrolyte imbalance)
    - Head trauma
    - Pneumonia
  - The first indication of decreased systemic perfusion is altered level of consciousness.

- How does the patient's age affect your assessment approach?
  - You decide to augment your assessment approach with GEMS components due to the patient's age.
  - Keep in mind that AMS in a geriatric patient is nonspecific.

The scene appears safe as you don your PPE while approaching the house. You are met at the door by the patient's wife who tells you the patient "isn't acting like himself." He is in an upstairs bedroom, lying in bed. On the way to the patient, you note that the residence is well-kept and without significant obstacles. The temperature in the house is warm. The wife appears supportive and concerned. While leading you to the patient, the wife tells you that the patient suddenly became confused and his behavior is not normal. She states he had a fall earlier today at his doctor's office. He was taken by EMS to the hospital where he was assessed and released.

As you reach the bedroom door, she mentions that they live together and receive no outside help. Their family all live some distance away, rarely visit, and are unable to help. She called 911 for transport to the hospital because she could not get him downstairs to the car to go back to the hospital this afternoon.

You enter the bedroom and see the patient lying in bed and uneaten food on the nightstand. The patient appears agitated and restless, is pale, and is breathing fast.

QUESTIONS

- Do you have any concerns based on your findings so far?
  - AMS is always a concern, especially in a geriatric patient. Rapid breathing may indicate respiratory distress. Pale skin suggests poor perfusion.

You perform a primary survey, which reveals:

- X–No observable bleeding noted.
- A–Patent airway.
- B–Breathing is fast and shallow with clear lung sounds bilaterally when auscultated.
- C–Radial pulse is fast and irregular. His skin is pale, warm, and clammy to the touch.
- D–He is alert and oriented to self and place only; pupils are PERRL.
- E–On exposure there are no signs of trauma, rash, or edema.

QUESTIONS

- What is the cardinal presentation and the chief complaint?
  - Cardinal presentation is the patient's medical problem: AMS (confusion)
  - Chief complaint is what the patient complains of: N/A in this case.

- Are any interventions required before assessment can continue?
  - No

- Does this patient require immediate transport, or can you remain on scene and continue your assessment?
  - You decide it is safe to remain on scene and continue your assessment.

- Has your differential diagnosis changed?
  - You rule out pneumonia, but the rest remains the same at this time.

- What further assessments would you like to perform?
  - Besides a detailed history, vital signs and physical assessment, you also ask the patient key questions for determining altered mental status.

The patient can communicate, but rambles and cannot stay on topic, so the OPQRST assessment of the chief complaint is limited:

- O–Sudden onset
- P–No pain, but has disordered thoughts
- Q–Has a sensation of paranoia and excitement
- R–Complaint is limited to thought disturbance, no weakness or altered sensation
- S–Distracted thought is 10/10
- T–1 hour

Altered Mental Status: Key Questions

- Was the patient exposed to alcohol, drugs, or toxins?
  - Patient is on nine prescription medications

- What is the patient normally like?
  - Normally independent and able to perform activities of daily living, A&O × 4

- When was the last time the patient was noted as having their baseline mental status?
  - Approximately 1 hour ago

- Did the patient complain of headache, or does the patient have a headache now?
  - No headache

- Did the patient have a preceding infection?
  - No

- Did or does the patient have a fever?
  - No

- Has the patient had any falls?
  - Yes, fell from standing to tile floor early this morning at doctor's office

- Is the patient feeling ill in any way?
  - Feels anxious and unable to control thoughts

- Is the patient adequately nourished?
  - Wife reports patient has had decreased appetite over 3 days

- Has the patient complained of neck stiffness?
  - No

- Presence of a body rash?
  - No

A SAMPLER history is also collected from the patient's wife:

- S–Agitation, confusion, rambling thoughts
- A–There are no known allergies
- M–He is compliant with prescriptions of aspirin, amitriptyline, clonazepam, digoxin, diphenhydramine, levothyroxine, losartan, omeprazole, and trazodone
- P–Atrial fibrillation, peptic ulcer, hypothyroidism, hypertension, sleep disorder
- L–Last meal was breakfast; patient has had decreased appetite and refuses to drink liquids

- E–Fall earlier today; had physical examination, lab work, and CT scan at hospital following fall with no injuries or abnormalities found
- R–Age, heart arrythmia, polypharmacy, fall

While you are collecting the patient's history from his wife, your partner assesses the following vital signs:

- HR: 78, irregular
- RR: 24
- BP: 128/84
- SpO$_2$: 97% room air
- ETCO$_2$: 32 mm Hg
- Temp: 98.7°F (37°C)
- 12-lead ECG N/A (patient is too agitated to obtain)
- BG: 122 mg/dl (6.8 mmol/l)
- GCS: 14 (E4, V4, M6)

Prior to placing the patient on your stretcher, you conduct a head-to-toe physical exam, which is unremarkable.

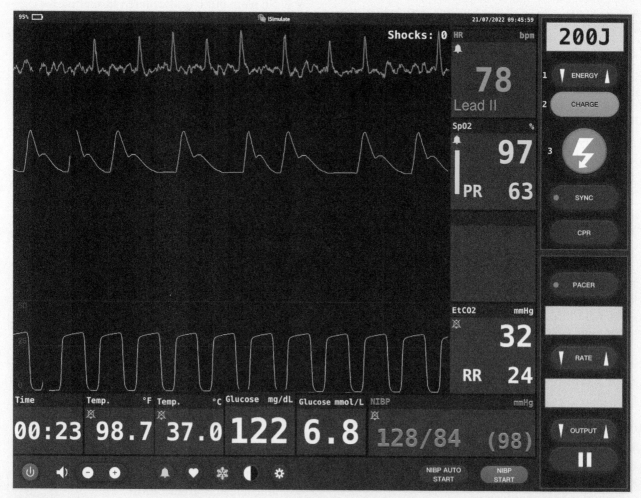

FIGURE 7-7

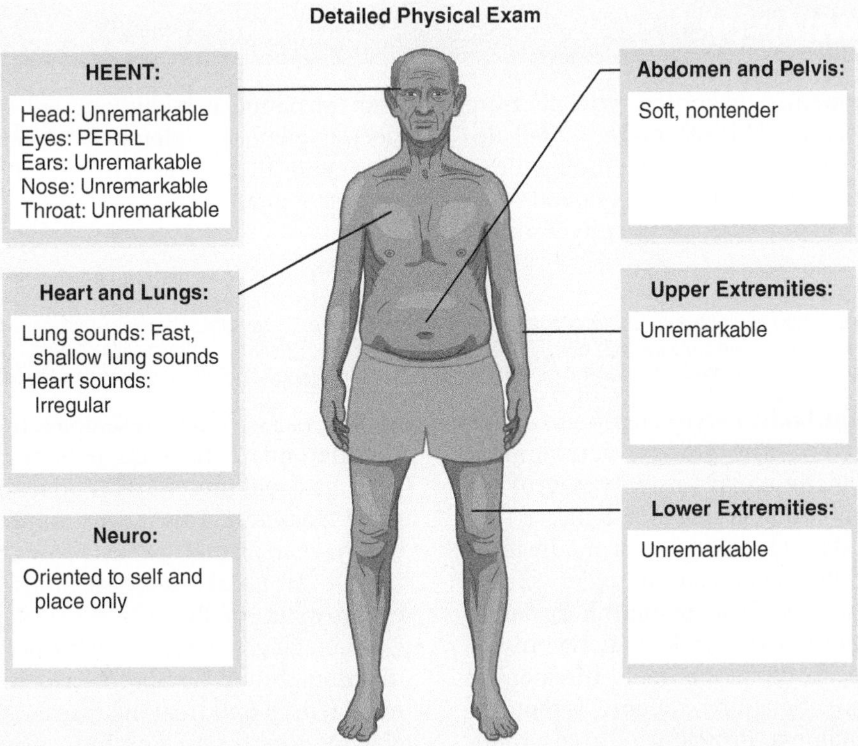

Detailed Physical Exam

HEENT:
Head: Unremarkable
Eyes: PERRL
Ears: Unremarkable
Nose: Unremarkable
Throat: Unremarkable

Heart and Lungs:
Lung sounds: Fast,
  shallow lung sounds
Heart sounds:
  Irregular

Neuro:
Oriented to self and
  place only

Abdomen and Pelvis:
Soft, nontender

Upper Extremities:
Unremarkable

Lower Extremities:
Unremarkable

FIGURE 7-8

QUESTIONS

- What does your differential diagnosis include now?
  - Stroke
  - Hyperglycemia
  - Dehydration
  - Infection/sepsis

- What is your goal for prehospital treatment?
  - Patient is currently stable, but should be continuously monitored to ensure no deterioration during transport. Provide supportive care and reassurance to try to calm the patient.

- Where is the most appropriate treatment destination for this patient?
  - This patient should be transported to the closest appropriate facility.

GEMS DIAMOND REVIEW

How was the GEMS Diamond information applied in this case?

Geriatric Assessment: The patient is an 81-year-old male who is living independently with his wife.

Environmental Assessment: Home is well-kept, without significant obstacles. No assistive devices are present or being used. The patient appears to have appropriate food and needed supplies in the house. Temperature in the house is warm.

Medical Assessment: In addition to your findings from the detailed assessment and vital signs, the wife advises that she ensures he is compliant with his medications and all medical appointments.

Social Assessment: The patient can accomplish ADLs by himself with his wife's support. Both adult children live out of state.

You move the patient to the stretcher and place him in a position of comfort. You continuously calm and reassure the patient en route to hospital, but his level of anxiety and restlessness is unchanged on arrival at the ED.

On arrival at the ED, a Foley catheter was placed, lab samples were collected, and a CT scan was repeated and compared to the image taken earlier. The diagnosis of no traumatic injury was confirmed. A comprehensive neurologic exam was performed on the patient.

CASE STUDY WRAP-UP

The patient is subsequently diagnosed with delirium likely due to a combination of his age, his recent fall, dehydration, and multiple medications that are high risk for delirium. The patient is admitted to a general ward and his amitriptyline, clonazepam, diphenhydramine, and trazodone prescriptions are discontinued. Proper sleep hygiene is implemented for him while in the hospital, and after 5 days, his symptoms resolve and he returns home.

CHAPTER WRAP-UP

Unlike other cells in the body, nerve cells do not divide and replicate themselves. The gradual deterioration of these cells over a lifetime explains why neurologic complaints are so common in geriatric patients.

Epilepsy/seizures, stroke, and dementia are the most common neurologic disorders seen in older adults. Any patient who presents with acute neurologic deficit should be evaluated for stroke. Stroke may be present with mild and nonspecific symptoms or life-threatening and obvious symptoms. For some patients, symptoms as mild as vague numbness, dizziness, blurred vision, or a clumsy hand may be symptomatic of a stroke.

Delirium is often confused with dementia. Delirium has a sudden onset and resolves once the cause is treated. Dementia is a permanent loss of mental capacity. Recall that, although dementia progresses gradually and is associated with older adults, it is not part of the normal aging process.

Bell palsy closely resembles the signs of a stroke. To differentiate, have the patient raise their eyebrows. Bell palsy will present with upper and lower unilateral facial weakness. This means that the Bell palsy patient will have asymmetrical eyebrow raise. Stroke patients have lower facial muscle weakness and can move their eyebrows normally.

Managing patients with suspected neurologic dysfunction should be approached in a systematic manner. Identify and treat life threats. Consider differential diagnoses early based on history and physical findings, remembering that geriatric patients will present atypically. Neurologic assessment should be thorough to ensure subtle findings are identified.

AEIOU-TIPS, SNOT, and 4S are useful mnemonics for recalling causes of acute and chronic altered mental status.

REFERENCES

Albert M, Knoefel J. *Clinical Neurology of Aging*. 3rd ed. New York: Oxford University Press; 2011.

Aroor S, Singh R, Goldstein LB. BE-FAST (Balance, Eyes, Face, Arm, Speech, Time). *Stroke*. 2017;48(2):479–481. doi:10.1161/strokeaha.116.015169

Bleakley G, Cole M. Recognition and management of sepsis: the nurse's role. *Br J Nurs*. 2020;29(21):1248–1251. doi:10.12968/bjon.2020.29.21.1248

Center for Disease Control and Prevention. About Shingles (Herpes Zoster). https://www.cdc.gov/shingles/about/index.html. Updated June 26, 2019. Accessed May 5, 2021.

Center for Neurological Treatment & Research. Bell's Palsy Overview. http://www.neurocntr.com/bells-palsy.php. Published 2014. Accessed May 5, 2021.

Centers for Disease Control and Prevention. Epilepsy and Seizures. Last updated September 2020. Accessed on May 21, 2022.

Dellinger R, Levy M, Rhodes A, et al. Surviving sepsis campaign: international guidelines for management of severe sepsis and septic shock, 2012. *Crit Care Med*. 2013 Feb;41(2):580–637.

Guneysel O, Onultan O, Onur O. Parkinson's disease and the frequent reasons for emergency admission. *Neuropsychiatri Dis Treat*. 2008 Aug;4(4):711–714. doi:10.2147/ndt.s3007

Homann B, Plaschg A, Grundner M, et al. The impact of neurological disorders on the risk for falls in the community dwelling elderly: a case-controlled study. *BMJ Open*. 2013;3(11):e003367. doi:10.1136/bmjopen-2013-003367

Johns Hopkins Medicine. Bell's Palsy. https://www.hopkinsmedicine.org/health/conditions-and-diseases/bells-palsy. Published 2021. Accessed May 5, 2021.

Ladha E, House-Kokan M, Gillespie M. The ABCCs of sepsis: a framework for understanding the pathophysiology of sepsis. *CJCCN*. 2019;30(4):12–21.

Liu S, Yu W, Lü Y. The causes of new-onset epilepsy and seizures in the elderly. *Neuropsychiatr Dis Treat*. 2016;12:1425–1434. doi:10.2147/NDT.S107905

Lui SK, Nguyen MH. Elderly stroke rehabilitation: overcoming the complications and its associated challenges. *Curr Gerontol Geriatr Res*. 2018;2018:1–9. doi:10.1155/2018/9853837

ayo Clinic. Peripheral neuropathy. https://www.mayoclinic.org/diseases-conditions/peripheral-neuropathy/symptoms-causes/syc-20352061. Published July 3, 2021. Accessed May 5, 2021.

ayo Clinic. Shingles. https://www.mayoclinic.org/diseases-conditions/shingles/symptoms-causes/syc-20353054. Published September 7, 2021. Accessed October 22, 2021.

edscape. Septic Shock Treatment & Management. https://emedicine.medscape.com/article/168402-treatment. Updated October 7, 2020. Accessed May 5, 2021.

ational Association of Emergency Medical Technicians. *AMLS: Advanced Medical Life Support: An Assessment-Based Approach.* 3rd ed. Burlington, MA: Jones & Bartlett Learning; 2021.

ational Institute of Neurological Disorders and Stroke. *Peripheral Neuropathy Fact Sheet.* https://www.ninds.nih.gov/Disorders/Patient-Caregiver-Education/Fact-Sheets/Peripheral-Neuropathy-Fact-Sheet. Reviewed March 16, 2020. Accessed May 5, 2021.

Brien JM, Ali NA, Aberegg SK, Abraham E. Sepsis. *Am J Med.* 2007;120(12):1012–1022.

arkinson's Foundation. What is Parkinson's? https://www.parkinson.org/understanding-parkinsons/what-is-parkinsons. Published 2021. Accessed September 17, 2021.

emick DG. Pathophysiology of sepsis. *Am J Path.* 2007;170(5):1435–1444.

Sullivan B. Sepsis: 10 things you need to know to save lives. EMS1. https://www.ems1.com/sponsored-article/articles/sepsis-10-things-you-need-to-know-to-save-lives-CwhpS0ttm2FRrVty/. Published June 9, 2015. Accessed May 5, 2021.

Vidale S, Arnaboldi M, Frangi L, Longoni M, Monza G, Agostoni E. The large artery intracranial occlusion stroke scale: a new tool with high accuracy in predicting large vessel occlusion. *Front Neurol.* 2019 Feb;10:130.

Wester AL, Dunlop O, Melby KK, Dahle UR, Wyller TB. Age-related differences in symptoms, diagnosis, and prognosis of bacteremia. *BMC Infect Dis.* 2013 July;13:346.

World Health Organization. Neurological disorders public health challenges. https://www.who.int/mental_health/neurology/neurological_disorders_report_web.pdf. Published 2006. Accessed May 5, 2021.

World Health Organization. Sepsis. https://www.who.int/health-topics/sepsis#tab=tab_1. Published 2021. Accessed May 5, 2021.

Xiao H, Wang Y-X, Xu T, et al. Evaluation and treatment of altered mental status patients in the emergency department: life in the fast lane. *World J Emerg Med.* 2012;3(4):270–277. doi:10.5847/wjem.j.issn.1920-8642.2012.04.006

CHAPTER 8

Elder Maltreatment and Psychosocial Emergencies

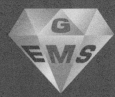

LESSON OBJECTIVES

- Discuss elder abuse, maltreatment, and neglect.
- Describe signs and symptoms of elder abuse, maltreatment, and neglect.
- Identify the profiles of an at-risk abuser and victim of elder abuse.

- Discuss the proper documentation and reporting of elder abuse.
- Review the epidemiology of depression, suicide, and substance abuse in the aging population.

Introduction

Elder abuse and neglect are extremely common, both in the home and community care settings. According to both U.S. and international studies, the estimated percentage of victims is thought to be much higher than currently known because maltreatment is primarily self-reported. Current self-reported ranges of any form of elder maltreatment, regardless of setting, are 2.4% to upwards of 10%, and rates vary widely based on location and type of maltreatment.

The type of maltreatment also plays a factor in prevalence. In a study published in 2017 by the *New England Journal of Medicine,* approximately 10% of older adults not in a community setting are victims of abuse or neglect. In an international study, half of community care workers admitted to elder maltreatment. Psychological abuse is reported most often, followed by financial abuse, neglect, physical abuse, and sexual abuse (**FIGURE 8-1**). An estimated 1 in 6 older adults worldwide are affected, or 15.7%.

Critical Thinking Question

Why are older adults more at risk of death due to abuse?

Elder Maltreatment

There are five general types of elder maltreatment, though a consensus in the worldwide medical community on definitions and types has not been reached. In **TABLE 8-1**, these types are listed in order of most to least prevalent.

A Growing Abuse Problem

According to one meta-analysis of elder maltreatment studies, elder abuse victims are expected to rise to 330 million worldwide by 2050.

Patterns have been identified in the characteristics of both the abuser and the abused. The geriatric person being abused is likely to live with the abuser, be socially isolated due to loss or inability to visit friends and relatives, or have increased needs due to mental or physical impairment. The abuser of a geriatric person is likely to live with their victim, be financially dependent on the victim, be under pressure due to work constraints, be socially isolated due to pressures of caregiving, have a history of poor family relationships, have a mental disorder, or suffer an addiction to alcohol or other substances.

Many tools have been developed to globally screen for elder abuse, but their efficacy has been limited due to variations in legal definitions of elder abuse and cultural differences.

TABLE 8-1 Types of Elder Mistreatment	
Maltreatment Type	Description
Psychological	Verbal abuse, threats, infantilizing, intimidation, deprivation of sensory stimulation, isolation (FIGURE 8-1)
Financial	Theft of valuables, improper use of guardianship or power of attorney
Neglect	Not providing essentials for life such as nutrition, personal hygiene, and maintaining a safe personal environment
Physical	Physical force resulting in bodily injury, force-feeding, administering chemical restraint
Sexual	Nonconsensual sexual contact or any sexual interaction with an elderly person lacking the capacity to give consent

Copyright © 2024 National Association of Emergency Medical Technicians (NAEMT).

Maltreatment in Long-Term Care Facilities

Maltreatment rates are higher in long-term care and community facilities such as nursing homes, rehabilitation centers, and assisted living facilities, as compared to society in general. The most common type of institution-related maltreatment is psychological, with staff admitting to calling patients names or threatening to harm them (FIGURE 8-2). The second most common form is neglect. Neglect can include letting the patient wait for care, such as toileting needs, or removing food before the patient is finished eating. Other reported maltreatment includes physical and sexual abuse.

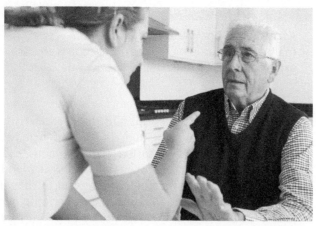

FIGURE 8-1 Psychological abuse of older adults is the most common and most often reported type of abuse. Verbal abuse, threats, and intimidation are all types of psychological abuse.
© SpeedKingz/Shutterstock

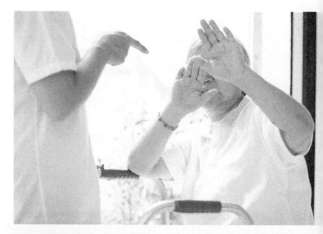

FIGURE 8-2 Maltreatment rates are higher in long-term care facilities such as nursing homes, rehabilitation centers, and assisted-living facilities.
© CGN089/Shutterstock

Long-term care residents who do not have visitors have a higher likelihood of being abused than those who do. Approximately 5% of the geriatric population in the United States lives in long-term care facilities and many do not receive visitors.

Characteristics associated with long-term care maltreatment can be categorized as physical or facility related. Evidence of physical maltreatment can include untreated injuries like pressure sores (**FIGURE 8-3**), broken bones, multiple wounds in various stages of healing, poor hygiene, malnourishment, family and friends complaining about poor level of care, torn or stained clothing, rashes or blisters to the perineal region, unmaintained medical devices such as overly filled urine collection bags, frequent need to consult or transport to hospital, and staff not following medical orders.

Facility-related maltreatment includes inadequate housekeeping practice, foul odors, not resolving problems when identified, and food left on trays in the dining areas. Indications of possible maltreatment and abuse can also include inconsistencies in staff reports, in medical records, or between staff and family statements. Staff may follow you during your assessment and monitor too closely, may have limited knowledge of the patient, or may be unwilling to release medical records.

Signs of Elder Maltreatment

Patients who are experiencing maltreatment at home may share similar characteristics to those in long-term care facilities, such as providing inconsistent history or having injuries inconsistent with the mechanism of injury provided (**FIGURE 8-4**). Detailed answers are best solicited by asking open-ended questions. When collecting history of events from a patient you suspect may be experiencing maltreatment, all information you obtain should be documented verbatim.

Physical signs of elder maltreatment in the home include signs like those associated with institutional maltreatment. Interactions between patient and caregiver should be carefully observed for anything unusual, such as the patient seemingly over-dependent on the caregiver or anxiety or depression without a medical or organic cause.

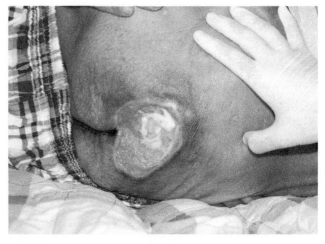

FIGURE 8-3 Pressure sore from neglect.
© phichet chaiyabin/Shutterstock

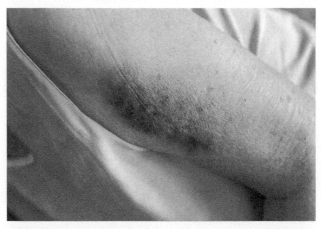

FIGURE 8-4 Bruising on the arm can be a sign of abuse, but detailed questioning of the patient must occur to determine the cause of physical injuries.
© KorArkaR/Shutterstock

Unless maltreatment is witnessed, evidence of abuse can only lead you to suspect that maltreatment has occurred. You are legally responsible to act on suspicion of maltreatment as if you had directly witnessed it.

Caregiver Stress

Caregiver stress, also known as **caregiver fatigue**, can lead to caregiver burnout. Although burnout can be a contributing factor for abuse, current research has found that elder abuse shares the same power and control dynamics as abuse of non-elderly persons.

The experience of caregiver stress is often underestimated by those who are caregivers, as their focus is on the caring of others rather than themselves. Risk factors for developing caretaker stress include living with the person receiving care, social isolation due to caregiving demand, depression or other mental health issues, financial difficulties, lack of down time to relax and focus on self, lack of coping skills to release stress, difficulty solving daily problems, lack of choice to take on role of caregiver, and caregivers that work outside their home.

If you suspect caregiver burnout, provide resources for the caregiver to receive support, such as access to support groups in your area, a reading list, and list of websites with useful information on how to relieve caregiver burnout.

Mental Health Disorders

Depression

Depression affects approximately 7 million older adult patients in the United States. This disorder affects women more than men and is more prevalent in long-term care facilities, where up to approximately 42% of residents are affected.

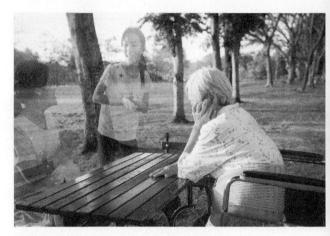

FIGURE 8-5 Social withdrawal, flattened mood, and decreased desire to participate in previously enjoyed activities are all signs and symptoms of depression.
© CGN089/Shutterstock

> ### Depression in Older Adults
>
> Depression is the most common psychiatric disorder among older adults in the United States.

With aging, a range of comorbidities, medications with adverse effects and interactions, increasing social isolation due to loss of family and friends, and decreasing physical functionality with its associated loss of independence all contribute heavily to the development of depression.

The American Psychological Association lists the following as common signs and symptoms of depression:

- Flattened mood
- Decreased interest or pleasure in doing activities previously enjoyed
- Substantial weight change
- Sleep disorder
- Physical immobility
- Easily agitated
- Lack of energy
- Feelings of worthlessness
- Decreased ability to concentrate or think
- Thoughts of suicide

Behaviors that are associated with depression are frequent, nonemergent calls for EMS; frequent ED or doctor office visits; poor personal hygiene; unkept home; withdrawal from social network (**FIGURE 8-5**); and complaint severity that is inconsistent with clinical findings.

Prehospital care practitioners should not provide counseling in an attempt to help the patient. Prehospital care should be limited to listening to the patient while transporting the patient to a hospital with psychiatric capabilities if a hospital level of care is indicated.

Suicide

The rate of suicide in the older adult population is thought to be underreported. Approximately 50% of suicides are classified as accidental, natural causes, or traumatic in nature. The statistics indicate that older adult males are seven times more likely to die by suicide than older adult females.

In younger age groups, suicide attempts are often impulsive and arise situationally, often due to unresolved concerns or other underlying issues that are not being addressed. In older adults, suicide attempts often have been considered for a length of time; they are well-planned and highly lethal. The high lethality of suicide in older adults is due to the following factors: methods of suicide selected, increased physical fragility,

> ### Suicide in Older Adults
>
> The older adult population in almost all industrialized countries has the highest rate of death by suicide compared to all other age groups. The top three suicide methods chosen by older adults are:
>
> - Firearms
> - Poisoning
> - Suffocation

isolation leading to decreased chances of interruptions and being found too late, and little to no warning of intent.

Lifestyle-related factors can increase the risk of an older adult considering suicide. Older adults with loss of mobility often feel isolated, have lower self-esteem, and lack a sense of well-being. Additionally, loss of independence often leads to economic insecurities and a sense of loss of control. Similar feelings can also occur with substantial loss of roles in life, such as retirement, which may contribute to a lack of purpose and sense of hopelessness.

Medical-related factors can also increase the risk of suicidal ideation. Comorbidities and medications often affect mentation. Medical history, current prescriptions, and recent changes to prescriptions must also be investigated as potential causes for suicidal thoughts.

Situational factors such as death of a spouse, friend, or family member also increase the risk of suicide.

Alcohol Dependence and Suicide

Studies show that persons with an alcohol dependence disorder are 50% to 70% more likely to die by suicide.

EMS practitioners should be vigilant in looking for warning signs of suicide. The IS PATH WARM mnemonic shown in **TABLE 8-2** can be used as a reminder for potential risk factors for suicidal thoughts.

TABLE 8-2 IS PATH WARM

Mnemonic	Factor
I	Ideation
S	Substance abuse
P	Purposelessness
A	Anxiety
T	Trapped
H	Hopelessness
W	Withdrawal
A	Anger
R	Recklessness
M	Mood change

Substance Abuse

According the Substance Abuse and Mental Health Services Administration (SAMHSA), nearly 1 million adults aged 65 and older in the United States live with a substance use disorder (SUD), as reported in 2018 data. Substance abuse in older adults can be deliberate (taking too much of a prescription medication, overuse of additive drugs) or accidental (inadvertently taking too much of a drug). In this age group, deliberate substance abuse can occur through prescription medications, legal substances (i.e., alcohol or marijuana), or illicit substances. Accidental abuse of a medication is covered in Chapter 2: Polypharmacy and Toxicity in Older Patients.

Over-the-counter and prescription medication abuse and misuse are the most common forms of substance abuse in the geriatric population. Abuse may result from:

- The misunderstanding that taking extra medication will resolve symptoms more quickly
- Stopping prescriptions when symptoms resolve without consulting a physician
- Using old medications or medications prescribed to another in order to avoid waste or to save money

Alcohol overuse is also very common (**FIGURE 8-6**). There are many contributing factors that lead to alcohol dependence in the geriatric population. These can include depression, chronic physical illness, chronic pain, job loss, and loss of financial resources. Alcohol is often used to suppress anxiety associated with changing from a busy lifestyle to the boredom of retirement.

Signs and symptoms of substance abuse can include those of depression and medication toxicity discussed in Chapter 2.

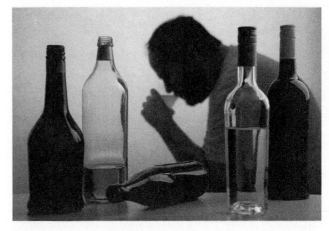

FIGURE 8-6 Alcohol overuse is common and may be used to suppress anxiety or depression.
© Axel Bueckert/Shutterstock

Mental Health Emergency

The management of a patient experiencing a mental health emergency requires a specific treatment plan that addresses the underlying cause(s) of the emergency and not just the emergency itself. EMS practitioners must understand the importance of ensuring that patients are transferred to further care, either by transport or referral, to ensure that they receive the full care they require.

The incorporation of the GEMS Diamond in your geriatric assessment is critical in managing psychosocial emergencies, as it reminds EMS personnel of the need to evaluate the extent of the emergency and consider the underlying cause in geriatric patients. Remember, we are advocates for our patients and should keep their best interests in mind.

CASE STUDY

It is 1700 on a cold winter evening; air temperature is 50°F (10°C). You and your partner are staffing an emergency response ambulance and are dispatched to a long-term care facility for a 77-year-old male in respiratory distress.

QUESTIONS

- What is your differential diagnosis?
  - Respiratory distress is a nonspecific complaint, so the differential diagnosis covers a wide range:
    - Asthma
    - COPD
    - COVID-19
    - Pneumonia
    - Seasonal influenza
    - Heart failure
    - Allergic reaction
    - Anxiety
    - Trauma

- How does the patient's age affect your assessment approach?
  - You decide to augment your assessment approach with GEMS components due to the patient's age.

- What equipment should you bring with you to your patient's side?
  - Because the patient's complaint is nonspecific, you decide to bring in your monitor/defibrillator, ALS bag, suction, and oxygen

The scene appears safe as you don your PPE while approaching the facility. You are met at the door by a staff nursing aide who hands you patient transfer documentation and asks you to follow her to the patient's room. The nursing aide appears anxious. You note that the facility is tidy, clean, warm, well lit, free from odors, and without significant obstacles on the way to the patient. On the way to the room, she tells you that the patient has been a resident since his wife died 2 years ago. The patient's family all live some distance away

and visit every 6 to 8 weeks. It has been 9 weeks since their last visit and they are unable to help.

You enter the patient's room and see the patient standing against a wall. You note that a nurse and another nursing aide are holding the patient in place. The patient appears agitated and is breathing fast. He is dressed in torn and well-worn pajamas (**FIGURE 8-7**).

QUESTION

- Do you have any concerns based on your findings so far?
  - Elder abuse is suspected, but not directly observed.

- What is your differential diagnosis after your initial impression?
  - Asthma
  - COPD
  - COVID-19
  - Pneumonia
  - Seasonal influenza
  - Heart failure

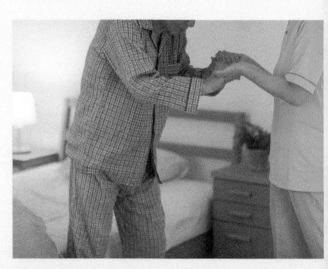

FIGURE 8-7

© sukiyaki/Shutterstock

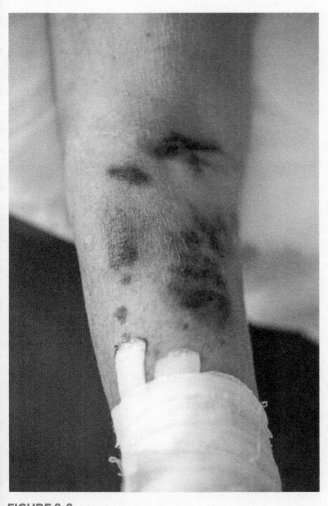

FIGURE 8-8
© Mironmax Studio/Shutterstock

- Allergic reaction
- Trauma
- Anxiety

You complete your primary survey, which reveals:

- X–No external bleeding noted.
- A–Airway is patent.
- B–Breathing seems adequate but is fast, rales are auscultated bilaterally at the lower lobes.
- C–Pulses are strong and regular; capillary refill is 3 seconds; skin is pale, cool, and clammy.
- D–Alert and restless; pupils are equal and reactive. GCS 14 (E4, V4, M6)
- E–On exposure no rashes are noted, but there is a large bruise at his left elbow (**FIGURE 8-8**).

QUESTIONS

- What is the cardinal presentation and the chief complaint?
  - Cardinal presentation: Respiratory distress
  - Chief complaint: Shortness of breath

- Are any interventions required before assessment can continue?
  - Not necessarily, but patient will benefit from:
    - Position of comfort
    - Oxygen
    - Bronchodilator

- Does this patient require immediate transport, or can you remain on scene and continue your assessment?
  - You decide it is safe to remain on scene and continue your assessment.

- Is this patient a possible victim of elder maltreatment?
  - There are enough signs to cause suspicion:
    - Unexplained bruise
    - Disheveled appearance

The patient is calmed and placed in the Fowler position on your stretcher. With some coaxing, he allows an oxygen mask to be placed and receives high-flow oxygen. You solicit your OPQRST and SAMPLER histories from the facility staff and the documentation handed to you.

The OPQRST:

- O–Sudden
- P–None
- Q–N/A
- R–None
- S–Unknown
- T–15 minutes

For more history, use the SAMPLER mnemonic.

- S–Dyspnea, agitation, bruise on left elbow
- A–No known allergies
- M–He is compliant with prescriptions of aspirin, ticagrelor, and captopril
- P–HF, MI (5 years previous), angioplasty with 2 stents (8 months previous)
- L–Last meal was this evening, 15 minutes before EMS call
- E–Dyspnea onset after eating dinner
- R–Age, heart disease, history of heart failure, does not know cause of bruising on left elbow

While you are collecting the patient's history, your partner assesses the following vital signs:

- HR: 110, regular
- RR: 24
- BP: 128/72
- SpO_2: 93% room air, improves to 98% with oxygen
- $ETCO_2$: 38 mm Hg
- Temp: 97.6°F (36.4°C)
- BG: 94 mg/dl (5.2 mmol/l)
- ECG sinus tachycardia
- 12-lead ECG pathologic Q waves in leads II, III, and aVF

You conduct a head-to-toe physical exam, which provides the following findings.

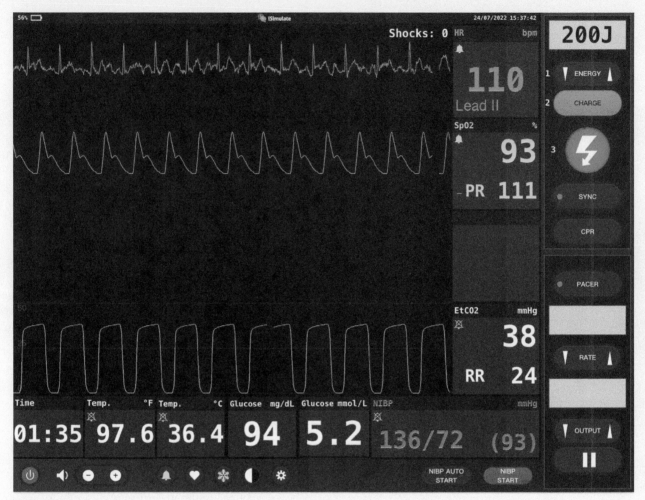

FIGURE 8-9

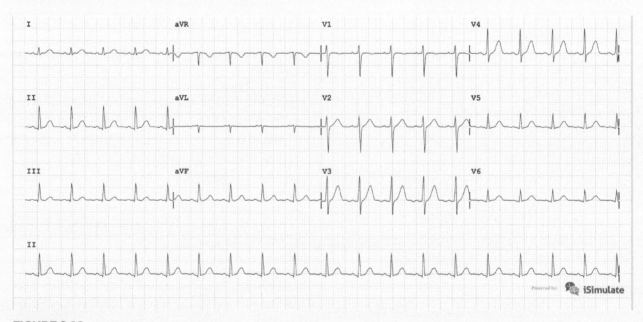

FIGURE 8-10

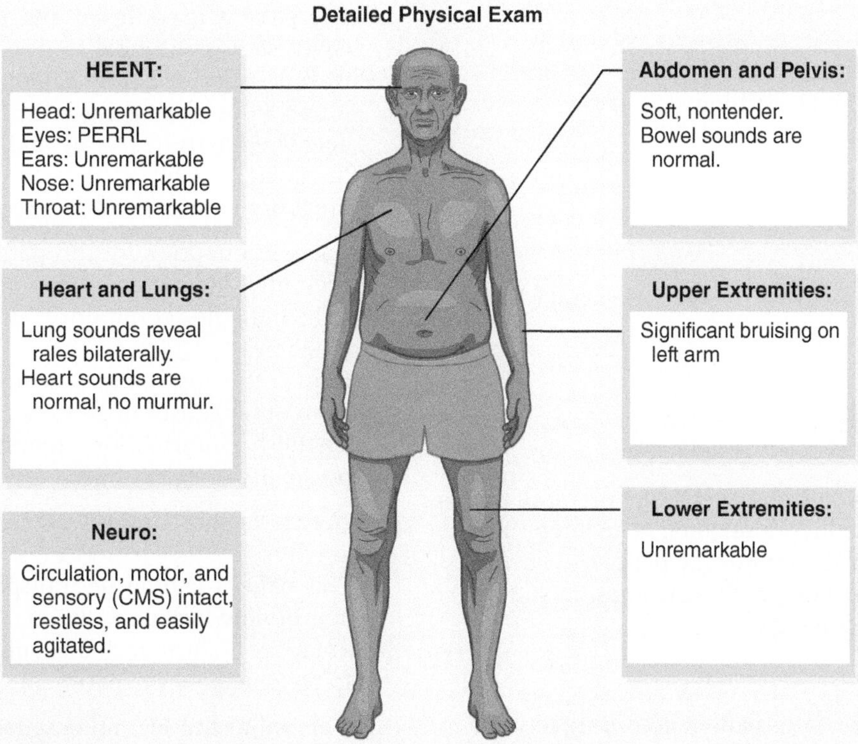

Detailed Physical Exam

HEENT:

Head: Unremarkable
Eyes: PERRL
Ears: Unremarkable
Nose: Unremarkable
Throat: Unremarkable

Heart and Lungs:

Lung sounds reveal
rales bilaterally.
Heart sounds are
normal, no murmur.

Neuro:

Circulation, motor, and
sensory (CMS) intact,
restless, and easily
agitated.

Abdomen and Pelvis:

Soft, nontender.
Bowel sounds are
normal.

Upper Extremities:

Significant bruising on
left arm

Lower Extremities:

Unremarkable

FIGURE 8-11

Copyright © 2024 National Association of Emergency Medical Technicians (NAEMT).

QUESTIONS

- Are there any abnormal findings? What might be causing these findings?
  - The patient's heart rate is tachycardic. This could be indicative of anxiety, heart failure, sepsis, or other infection.
- What does your differential diagnosis include now?
  - COVID-19
  - Pneumonia
  - Seasonal influenza
  - Heart failure
  - Anxiety
- What is your goal for prehospital treatment?
  - Treatment should be focused on supportive care and include:
    - Position of comfort
    - Oxygen
    - Bronchodilator

GEMS DIAMOND REVIEW

The GEMS Diamond review for this patient:

Geriatric Assessment: The patient is a 77-year-old male who requires some assistance with activities of daily living in an institutionalized setting. He has no dentures, hearing aids, or glasses, and is able to self-ambulate.

Environmental Assessment: Facility is well-kept, without significant obstacles. The patient appears to have appropriate food and needed supplies. Temperature in the room is warm and smells clean. Patient is wearing old and worn-out pajamas.

Medical Assessment: In addition to your findings from the detailed assessment and vital signs, the nurse advises you that the patient is compliant with his meds. A large bruise is noted at the patient's left elbow and staff is unsure of its cause.

Social Assessment: The patient can accomplish most ADLs by himself and receives support from staff with the rest. Patient's family lives some distance away and visits approximately every other month.

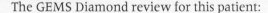

Treatment

- BLS
  - Monitor airway and breathing
  - Administer oxygen
  - Position of comfort
- ALS
  - BLS care
  - IV lock
  - Bronchodilator
  - Diuretic
- Critical care
  - BLS/ALS care
  - CPAP/BiPAP

As part of your ongoing management, you recall the importance of completing an ongoing assessment and reassess the patient. You monitor the patient to ensure interventions achieve therapeutic outcomes, including monitoring for adverse effects.

QUESTIONS

- How would you treat this patient according to your local protocols and scope of practice?
  - The patient should be treated with supportive care.
  - Be prepared for rapid deterioration.
  - You decide to treat your patient for exacerbation of HF. In addition to continuing oxygen therapy, you initiate an IV line and administer a loop diuretic.

The patient is confused and uncooperative with CPAP, so it is withheld.
  - During transport, the patient is reassessed and found to be improving as he is less anxious, has decreased both heart rate and breathing rate, and has increased bilateral air movement when the lungs are auscultated.

- What are your goals for this patient?
  - Promptly identify and manage the patient by reducing the respiratory distress to improve outcome.
  - Deliver the appropriate therapy by differentiating from other causes of geriatric respiratory distress.
  - Establish information required to determine possibility of elder abuse.

- Where is the most appropriate treatment destination and why?
  - This patient should be transported to the closest appropriate facility.
  - There are no further changes noted during transport to the emergency department.

On arrival at the ED, prehospital therapies are continued. The patient is now calm and compliant with instructions, so CPAP is applied and is well tolerated. Blood samples are taken for lab analysis and a chest x-ray is taken, which confirms HF, and also confirms no food was aspirated during his meal. You inform the ED physician of your concerns regarding the potential for elder abuse.

CASE STUDY WRAP-UP

The patient is admitted with the diagnosis of HF exacerbation. He is kept at the hospital for 2 days for observation and to allow time for the suspected elder abuse to be investigated. The dyspnea resolves within an hour of ED admission.

The investigation into elder abuse reveals that the patient is well cared for and has no complaints of the facility. His old pajamas are his favorite and most comfortable clothing, which he requested to wear. The bruise on his left elbow resulted from blood samples drawn by his doctor's clinic 3 days before the EMS call. The patient is returned to the long-term care facility following the investigation after 2 days in the hospital.

CHAPTER WRAP-UP

Knowing the risks and patterns of behavior associated with elder abuse will allow for early identification of suspected cases. Cases of abuse are more common in long-term care facilities where overwork, understaffing, and quality assurance lapses can allow general abuse to become tolerated and even normalized. In a home situation, elder abuse is primarily caused by power and control dynamics within the relationship between the caregiver and patient.

The management of a patient experiencing a mental health emergency requires a specific follow-up treatment plan that deals with the underlying causes of the emergency crisis that triggered an EMS response.

The incorporation of the GEMS Diamond in your geriatric assessment is necessary for managing psychosocial emergencies, as it can be an effective tool in identifying the root cause of the disorder. Managing the causative factors before a psychosocial disorder or abuse situation occurs is the optimal solution.

REFERENCES

Adult Protective Services Reporting Laws. American Bar Association Commission on Law and Aging. https://www.americanbar.org/content/dam/aba/administrative/law_aging/2020-elder-abuse-reporting-chart.pdf. Published April 2022. Accessed June 24, 2022.

Brandl B, Raymond J. Policy implications of recognizing that caregiver stress is not the primary cause of elder abuse. *Generations.* 2012;36(3):32–39.

Szanto K, Gildengers A, Mulsant BH, et al. Identification of suicidal ideation and prevention of suicidal behaviour in the elderly. *Drugs Aging.* 2002;19(1):11–24.

King KC, Goldstein S. Congestive heart failure and pulmonary edema. https://www.ncbi.nlm.nih.gov/books/NBK554557/. Updated September 21, 2021. Accessed March 22, 2021.

Lachs M, Pillemer K. Elder abuse. *N Engl J Med.* 2015;373:1947–1956.

Onega L. The Modified Caregiver Strain Index (MCSI). https://hign.org/sites/default/files/2020-06/Try_This_General_Assessment_14.pdf. Last reviewed 2018. Accessed March 24, 2021.

Substance Abuse and Mental Health Services Administration. Results from the 2018 National Survey on Drug Use and Health: Detailed tables. Rockville, MD: Center for Behavioral Health Statistics and Quality, Substance Abuse and Mental Health Services Administration. https://www.samhsa.gov/data/. Published 2019. Accessed September 22, 2022.

World Health Organization. Elder Abuse. https://www.who.int/news-room/fact-sheets/detail/elder-abuse. Published October 4, 2021. Accessed September 22, 2022.

Yon Y, Mikton CR, Gassoumis ZD, Wilber KH. Elder abuse prevalence in community settings: a systematic review and meta-analysis. *Lancet Glob Health.* 2017;5(2):e147–e156. doi:10.1016/s2214-109x(17)30006-2

CHAPTER 9

End-of-Life and Palliative Care

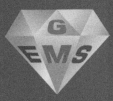

LESSON OBJECTIVES

- Differentiate between palliative and hospice care.
- Discuss legal end-of-life care documents as they relate to the care of the older patient.

- Identify the grieving and loss processes.
- Demonstrate the principles of effective communication with families and caregivers of deceased patients.

Introduction

In the 1980s, the World Health Organization recognized a need to better manage pain for cancer patients nearing the end of their lives. Since then, the end-of-life care concept has expanded to include any patient suffering from a chronic illness unresponsive to curative therapy. Care has also been extended beyond just pain relief and now includes the physical, emotional, and spiritual needs of the patient as well as those of the patient's family, friends, and caregivers.

This chapter is intended to review the concepts of palliative care and end-of-life treatments. Medical–legal documents and legalities of providing care discussed in the lesson pertain to the United States in general and may not be pertinent to your local jurisdiction. Refer to local statutes for legal guidance.

EMS professionals often witness death, and these events typically occur during a resuscitation attempt. The primary goals of EMS health care training involve promotion of health and prevention of death. Because of this focus, death may sometimes be viewed as a setback or failure, or an indication of incompetence on the part of the health care team. This perspective can cause coping difficulties because death can occur even when optimal care is provided perfectly. The inevitability of death is sometimes forgotten by health care practitioners who see their business as saving lives.

Top 11 Causes of Death in the United States (2020)

1. Heart disease
2. Cancer
3. COVID-19
4. Accident (unintentional)
5. Stroke
6. Chronic lower respiratory diseases
7. Alzheimer disease
8. Diabetes
9. Chronic liver disease and cirrhosis
10. Renal disease
11. Suicide

However, if the health care professional changes their goal from saving lives to providing the care needed by the patients, then comforting a dying patient through the death process may be more easily accepted (**FIGURE 9-1**).

Treat the Patient's Needs

The treatment goal is to provide the care the patient needs.

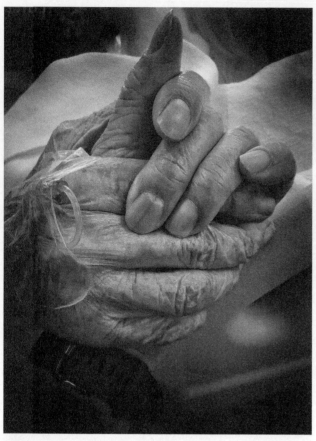

FIGURE 9-1 Comforting a dying patient is sometimes the care needed most.

© Ray's Images/Shutterstock

Cultural, religious, and personal views of death vary greatly. Some cultures and religions regard death as a sacred event, and being invited into the intimacy of a dying person's last moments is considered a privilege. In other cultures or belief systems, death is an emotionally traumatic event that must be avoided or delayed as long as possible and at whatever cost. Whatever the belief system, a patient's wishes for the care they receive must be respected. This is true at all stages of life, including how it ends. Every patient, their family, and their friends deserve our support and help in coping during this highly stressful and emotional time. Through experiencing the death of a patient, you should develop an understanding of how the stress associated with death and dying affects you.

Components of Compassionate Care

- Listen
- Communicate effectively
- Treat with compassion
- Respect patient's wishes

Listening and communicating effectively and with compassion are critical skills all health care personnel should develop and practice. This can be challenging when facing situations that conflict with you own personal beliefs. Respecting the patient's wishes and providing appropriate professional care may mean allowing your patient to die.

Palliative Care

Also known as "comfort care," **palliative care** focuses on treating the symptoms that can impact a patient's quality of life. The goal is to preserve a patient's day-to-day living and independence by reducing the severity of their symptoms. This differs from standard care in that there is no curative care provided. In other words, treatment goals revolve around making the patient as comfortable as possible instead of seeking a cure.

Although palliative care has been associated with end-of-life, it provides more benefit when it is started as soon as possible. It can be provided at any time and at any stage of an illness, whether a patient is terminal or not. It may even be provided concurrently with curative treatments, such as organ transplant or chemotherapy.

Palliative Care May Extend Life

Studies have shown that a patient's life expectancy is increased when palliative care is started early.

Comfort care could include patient positioning, hygiene, suctioning, oral care, analgesia, sedation, hydration, and environmental management such as adjusting room lighting, temperature, and air flow. Medications such as oxygen and antibiotics might be included as part of comfort care with the goal to make the patient more comfortable by alleviating or reversing symptoms. Comfort care does not involve invasive procedures such as establishing intravenous access or placing an advanced airway.

Hospice Care

Patients become eligible for hospice care when a physician determines that their life expectancy is 6 months or less, if their illness runs its normal course. By U.S. law, health care practitioners must certify that patients meet guidelines to be eligible for referral to a hospice provider.

The eligibility guidelines for hospice care require decline in functional status of at least one of the following:

Life expectancy is 6 months or less
Palliative Performance Scale (PPS) rating < 50%
- The Palliative Performance Scale is a tool used to assess the median number of days left before death. The tool uses five factors to rate on a scale from 0% to 100%. The lower the percentage, the less time expected before death.
Assistance required for at least three of the six activities of daily living.
Alteration in nutritional status such as > 10% loss of weight over last 6 months
Deterioration in overall condition during the last 6 months manifested by at least one of the following:
- Three or more hospitalizations or ED visits
- Decrease in tolerance to physical activity
- Decline in cognitive ability
- Other comorbid condition

In 2018, 1.55 million Americans entered hospice care. Hospice care can include home care, inpatient care, personalized care plans, supportive care to families, social worker assistance, chaplains, volunteers, and bereavement specialists. In most situations, a hospice care team is assigned to a hospice patient at the location best suited to the patient's needs (FIGURE 9-2). This can take place in the patient's home or in a hospice facility. If the patient chooses to die in a hospital, EMS may be called to transport the patient. Care during transport entails making the patient as comfortable as possible and, in the situation the patient dies, not attempting to resuscitate if proper, legally recognized documentation is with the patient.

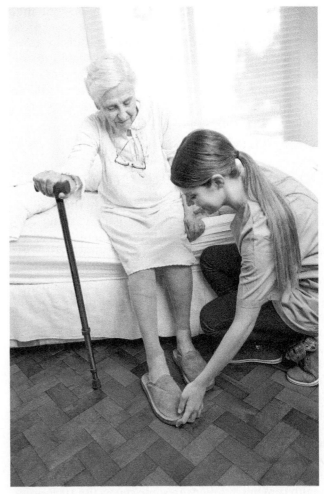

FIGURE 9-2 A member of a hospice care team helps a patient with dressing needs.
© Robert Kneschke/Shutterstock

Advance Directives

An **advance directive** is a written document that expresses the patient's wishes regarding their medical care. This document varies from jurisdiction to jurisdiction. It may also be referred to as a living will or health care directive. This document is intended to guide medical decision making when the patient is no longer able to communicate their wishes. A **medical power of attorney (MPOA)** is a similar legal document that assigns a person to make medical decisions on the patient's behalf when the patient is unable to express their desires. A **durable power of attorney (POA)** is similar to the MPOA as it can also designate a person to make medical decisions for the incapacitated patient. **Guardianship** is a directive by a court that declares someone incompetent and appoints another person to make decisions on their behalf. Guardianship can include health care decisions.

The medical care described in an advance directive will depend on how the patient wants to be treated and typically directs the use of pain management, nutrition, hydration, and resuscitation. Each document is unique and must be reviewed carefully before assuming the care of the patient. This document may also designate a surrogate decision maker who can make decisions for the patient when the patient is no longer able capable of doing so.

Better to Be Prepared

Initiating a discussion with the patient or their family regarding the preparation of an advance directive is difficult, but makes decisions easier when the time comes.

The patient and family need to understand that an advance directive allows the patient to express their values and desires about their end-of-life care. Advance directives should be made available to the family and health care practitioners in the event of an emergency. A copy of the advance directive should be kept with the patient, so it is available for EMS practitioners to consult prior to potentially initiating unwanted care.

Do Not Resuscitate Orders

Do not resuscitate (DNR) orders specify the medical care to be performed should the patient suffer cardiac arrest (**FIGURE 9-3**). This document is also referred to as Do Not Attempt Resuscitation (DNAR). DNRs/DNARs serve the same purpose and are used in identical situations. DNAR has been adopted in some jurisdictions to reflect the low success rate of resuscitation for these patients. Some jurisdictions have two types of DNR documents. An **in-hospital DNR** is included in the patient's medical file and is only valid while the patient is admitted to the hospital identified by the file. An **out-of-hospital DNR (OOH-DNR)** is intended for reference by EMS personnel.

To be valid, DNR and OOH-DNR orders must clearly state the patient's wish for resuscitative measures, must be signed by the patient or legal guardian, and must be signed by one or more physicians or other licensed health care practitioners. In some states, the DNR order must be dated and have an expiration date not to exceed 12 months from the signing date.

In many states, EMS can only honor a valid OOH-DNR document, while the other kinds of orders are for use in health care facilities.

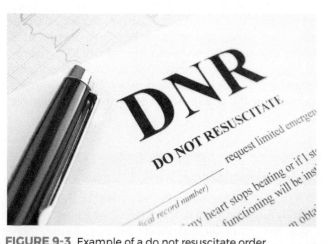

FIGURE 9-3 Example of a do not resuscitate order.
© Marc F Gutierrez/Shutterstock

Orders for Life-Sustaining Treatment

Medical orders for life-sustaining treatment (MOLST) or **physician orders for life-sustaining treatment (POLST)** explain medical care for the patient in the form of medical orders. This document must be signed by an authorized medical practitioner to be valid. Depending on the state, the authorized medical practitioner could be a nurse practitioner, physician assistant, or a physician.

The main difference between a MOLST or POLST and a DNR is that a MOLST or POLST can include a variety of end-of-life treatments, whereas a DNR order is restricted to care provided when a patient stops breathing or their heart stops beating.

Guidelines for these documents also vary by state but generally include the patient's right to refuse treatment if they can communicate. As these are newer documents, it is prudent to review state and local guidelines regarding MOLST/POLST.

> ### When in Doubt, Treat the Patient
>
> When in doubt of the validity of an advance directive or it is not present, you have the legal obligation to treat the patient as though the advance directive does not exist.

Bereavement, Grieving, and Mourning

Although bereavement, grieving, and mourning are often considered as synonymous, they each have their own meaning (**FIGURE 9-4**). **Mourning** is the process by which someone adapts to a death. The mourning process is unique to each person. **Grieving** is the process of emotional response to a death. This process typically follows a predictable pattern. **Bereavement** is the time or state of having a loss in which mourning and grieving occur after a death and often depends on the degree of attachment a person had to the deceased. Religious and cultural beliefs and rituals will have a significant effect on all three concepts.

A person's reaction to a terminal illness will vary and can range from openly discussing it to hiding or denying the illness. An expected instinct is to try to make the patient feel better by saying reassuring statements such as "Everything will be alright," or hopeful statements like "You can beat this." Making positive

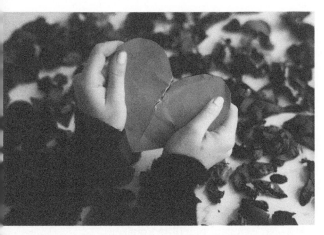

FIGURE 9-4 The processes of mourning, grieving, and bereavement are unique to each person following a death.
© Rawpixel.com/Shutterstock

TABLE 9-1 Phrases to Use and Avoid

Examples of Helpful Phrases to Use	Examples of Hurtful Phrases to Avoid
I'm so sorry for your loss.	They have gone to a better place.
I can't imagine how difficult this is for you.	Everything will be okay.
How can I help?	At least their suffering is over.
I imagine this is very painful for you.	It could have been worse.

Copyright © 2024 National Association of Emergency Medical Technicians (NAEMT).

statements may feel like a good approach, especially when you don't know what to say (**TABLE 9-1**). However, platitudes and promises that cannot be kept can further emotionally stress or even anger the patient.

The best strategy is to actively listen and allow the patient to voice their concerns, frustrations, or fears. Be prepared for emotions such as sadness, anger, or anxiety. Ask open-ended questions to encourage the patient to answer more freely. Keep the environment as quiet as possible as this reinforces a respectful tone for the patient. Not all patients will want to speak. You can always tell the patient that you don't know what to say (because there aren't always words for these situations), but you will listen, and/or you can also sit in silence with them and let them know you are truly there with them to offer comfort in whatever way possible. Silence together can often be solace.

When interacting with the family of a patient nearing the end of life, answer their questions honestly and in a way that they can understand. For instance, family members may be concerned when they witness Cheyne-Stokes respirations and think the patient is in distress. An explanation that this type of breathing is a normal part of the death process, and the patient does not feel discomfort, may be helpful.

EMS practitioners must understand their own set of beliefs and be prepared to respect the beliefs of others, as responses to death will vary greatly. Effective communication is key and helps determine the wishes of the patient and their family, allowing you to be as helpful as you can. Be aware of language barriers and how the patient or caregiver wishes to be greeted and spoken to. Allow the patient and family to be active participants if they wish to be.

Never Be Judgmental

Survivors will experience a range of feelings and grieve in their own way, which may be different from you or in a way you are unfamiliar with. There is no "correct" way to grieve, and all expressions of grief are valid.

CASE STUDY

You and your partner are working the night shift for an emergency ambulance service. You are dispatched to a long-term care facility for an 87-year-old female with shortness of breath. It is a chilly fall evening.

QUESTIONS

- What conditions are on your differential diagnosis list?
  - Shortness of breath is not specific, so it could be any number of illnesses or traumatic conditions.

You consider that it may also be an indication that a respiratory infection is spreading in the facility. Your differential diagnosis includes the following:
- COPD
- Lung cancer
- Heart failure
- COVID-19
- Asthma
- Anxiety

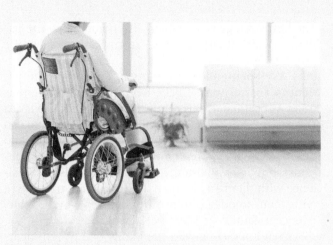

FIGURE 9-5

© sukiyaki/Shutterstock

- ◦ Infection—sepsis
- ◦ Pneumothorax
- ◦ Pulmonary embolism
- ◦ AMI
- ◦ Polypharmacy

- How does the patient's age affect your assessment approach?
  - You decide that you will include the GEMS approach to your assessment due to the patient's age. You also recall that in your area, long-term care patients are required to complete an advance directive when admitted. You note that you will need to determine the patient's wishes for her medical care when you first arrive.

- What equipment should you bring with you to your patient's side?
  - You decide to bring the stretcher, oxygen, med kit, and airway kit.

You arrive at the front entrance of the facility and are met by facility staff who lead you to the patient's room. The facility is clean, well lit, and has no odors, and the hallways are free of obstacles. When you get to the patient's room you find her awake and sitting in a recliner. Her breathing seems fast, but her skin is cyanosed. You notice that she has a nasal cannula in place, wears glasses, and uses a walker. There are stacks of newspapers and magazines cluttering the room, and the room feels cool. You assess that the scene is safe and you are wearing the correct PPE.

The facility nurse is standing beside the patient. He tells you that they check on the patient every hour and during this last check, he found the patient in her chair, short of breath, with her nasal cannula displaced from her nose. The nurse replaced her cannula and applied the oxygen at 2 lpm and assisted the patient to the recliner, where her SpO$_2$ remained at 88%. Because her oxygen saturation did not improve with reapplication

of the nasal cannula, the staff encouraged her to go t the hospital.

The nurse hands you a copy of the patient's healt information. You skim through the notes and find valid DNR and OOH-DNR and requests no heroic mea sures to be taken should she stop breathing.

The patient wishes that care be limited to pain re lief, passive oxygenation, and bleeding control. As yo communicate with the patient, you note that she ap pears to be hard of hearing; staff explains that she i supposed to wear hearing aids, but does not have an due to inability to pay for them.

You perform a primary survey and find the followin

- X–No external bleeding apparent
- A–Airway is patent
- B–Breathing is deep and faster than normal. Lung are auscultated and wheezes are heard bilaterally.
- C–Radial pulses are rapid, strong, regular; skin cool, dry, and cyanosed
- D–GCS is 15 (E4, V5, M6), pupils are 5 mm, equa and sluggish
- E–No wounds, rashes, or edema found

QUESTIONS

- What is the cardinal presentation and the chi complaint?
  - Cardinal presentation: Respiratory distress
  - Chief complaint: Shortness of breath

- Are any interventions required before assessmen can continue?
  - Following local protocols, you increase the oxyge flow to 6 lpm and, since wheezes are a reversib symptom, you administer an albuterol treatmen

- Does this patient require immediate transport, or ca you remain on scene and continue your assessment
  - After increasing oxygen flow, you decide you ca remain on scene and continue your assessment.

- What further assessments would you like to perform
  - Using the GEMS approach, you perform OPQRS and SAMPLER assessments, take the patient's vita signs, perform an ECG, and complete a physica head-to-toe assessment.

Your partner assesses vital signs while you consu the facility staff and medical notes for the OPQRST an SAMPLER assessments.

- O–Unknown, as patient was found short of breat during a routine check
- P–Lying supine makes shortness of breath worse
- Q–None
- R–None
- S–None
- T–60 minutes prior to being found SOB

- S–Shortness of breath
- A–Penicillin
- M–Staff state the patient is compliant with bevacizumab, metoprolol, atorvastatin, omeprazole, loratadine, gabapentin, acetaminophen, albuterol, prednisolone, oxygen at 2 lpm via nasal cannula; advance directive in place and with patient
- P–Hypertension, lung cancer, COPD, hyperlipidemia, GERD, hearing loss, and depression
- L–Ate a sandwich at lunch
- E–Facility staff said the patient has had a productive cough for several days and today her breathing seems much worse than normal. During a routine check she was found with shortness of breath and her nasal cannula was not in her nose
- R–Age, lung cancer, COPD, HTN, smoker for 45 years, polypharmacy

Her vital signs:

- HR: 110
- SpO$_2$: 88% on 2 lpm via NC
- RR: 24
- BP: 156/94
- Temp: 97.6°F (36.4°C)
- ETCO$_2$: 48 mm Hg
- BGL: 86 mg/dl (4.8 mmol/l)
- ECG shows sinus tachycardia
- 12-lead ECG is unremarkable

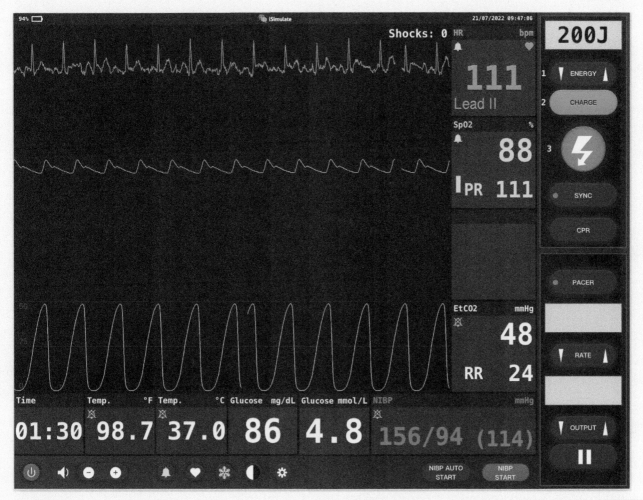

FIGURE 9-6

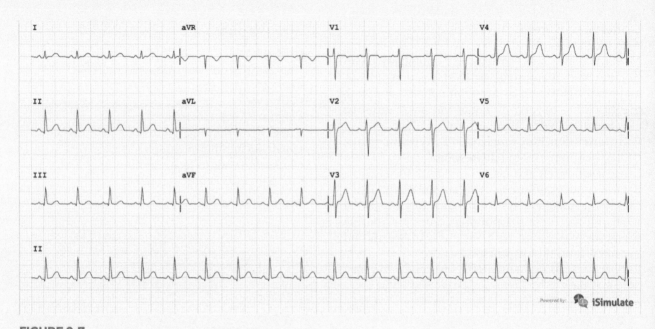

FIGURE 9-7

A physical head-to-toe assessment is performed and no new findings were noted.

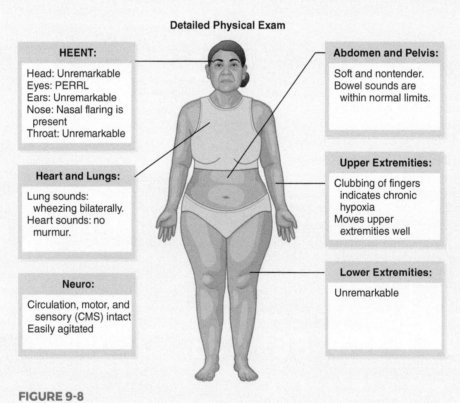

FIGURE 9-8

GEMS DIAMOND REVIEW

Geriatric Assessment: The patient has age-related changes expected for an 87-year-old.

Environmental Assessment: The room is cluttered; the staff reports that the room is kept cooler for the patient's comfort as warmer temperatures make it feel stuffier and harder to breathe.

Medical Assessment: Facility staff report the patient is compliant with medications and there have been no recent prescription changes. Patient has valid DNR/OOH-DNR, as well as directive to only provide pain relief, passive oxygenation, and bleeding control.

Social Assessment: The patient's husband died a year ago, and her family visits every few months. She is assisted with ADLs and receives her food from the facility.

QUESTIONS

- What does your differential diagnosis include now?
  - Exacerbation of COPD
  - Exacerbation of lung cancer
  - HF
  - Pneumonia
  - Anxiety
  - PE
  - Polypharmacy

- What are your goals for this patient?
  - The patient should be treated with supportive care.
  - Improve oxygenation
  - Monitor patient for any changes.
  - Deliver appropriate therapy.

- What treatment should be provided if the patient suddenly deteriorates and becomes bradycardic and apneic?
  - Because the patient had an OOH-DNR, it needs to be honored. Comfort care would continue, but no heroic measures should be used, such as RSI and placing her on a transport ventilator.

Your treatment includes:

- BLS
  - Position of comfort
  - Oxygen to improve saturations
  - Albuterol breathing treatment
  - Monitor vitals

- ALS
  - BLS care
  - BiPAP/CPAP

- Critical care
  - BLS/ALS care

She is transported in Fowler position and monitored throughout transport. Her SpO$_2$ improves to 94% with increased oxygen and albuterol treatment but her HR and RR remain unchanged. Wheezes are no longer heard when auscultating her lungs. The ambulance temperature is kept cool for the patient's comfort. There are no further changes noted during transport to the emergency department.

Her oxygen is continued at the hospital.

QUESTIONS

- Where is the most appropriate treatment destination and why?
  - This patient should be transported to the closest appropriate facility.

- What if the patient became bradycardic and apneic?
  - Because the patient had an OOH-DNR, it needs to be honored. Comfort care would continue, but no heroic measures should be used, such as RSI and placing her on a transport ventilator.

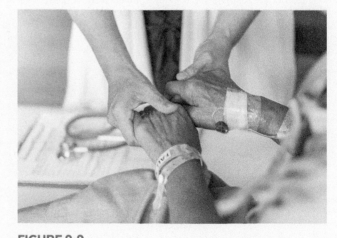

FIGURE 9-9

© Chinnapong/Shutterstock

CASE STUDY WRAP-UP

The patient is diagnosed with an upper respiratory infection that exacerbated her COPD and lung cancer. After consulting her OOH-DNR, the decision is made to not perform diagnostics and aggressively treat her. Because she is more comfortable at home than in an unfamiliar hospital setting, she is transported back to the long-term care facility with an increased oxygen prescription to 4 lpm of humidified oxygen by nasal cannula. Her other prescriptions are discontinued. Her mentation gradually deteriorates over the next 3 days; she dies on the fourth day with her family present.

CHAPTER WRAP-UP

Working with dying patients can be difficult as most people are not comfortable with their own mortality. Different belief systems deal with mortality in different ways and you may be expected to manage a patient whose beliefs contradict yours. Your role as a prehospital practitioner means that you must respect the patient's wishes within specific legal parameters despite any discomfort you have.

Effective listening and communication are critical skills the EMS practitioner must use with this type of patient interaction. Allow the time for the patient's family and friends to grieve and mourn their loss in their own way.

Advance directives allow the patient to receive the care they consent to when they are unable to speak for themselves. Be familiar with the advance directive legislation in the area in which you practice.

Remember that DNR does not mean do not treat. It only means that your ultimate goal of providing the best care for your patient now is limited to comfort care.

Allow time for family and friends for bereavement, grieving, and mourning the death of a loved one.

REFERENCES

Anderson F, Downing GM, Hill J, Casorso L, Lerch N. Palliative performance scale (PPS): a new tool. *J Palliat Care.* 1996 Spring;12(1):5–11. PMID: 8857241.

Brighton L, Bristowe K. Communication in palliative care: talking about the end of life, before the end of life. *Postgrad Med J.* 2016 Dec;92(1090):466–470. https://pmj.bmj.com/content/92/1090/466.short. Published online May 6, 2016. Accessed on June 5, 2022.

Hanlon P. The role of oxygen in palliative care. *Clinical, Home Care, Medicare and Medicaid, Therapy Devices.* https://rtmagazine.com/department-management/clinical/role-oxygen-palliative-care/. Updated June 7, 2015. Accessed May 30, 2022.

Rome R, Luminais HH, Bourgeois DA, Blais CM. The role of palliative care at the end of Life. *Ochsner J.* 2011;11(4):348–352.

Sepúlveda C, Martin A, Yoshida T, Ullrich A. Palliative care: the World Health Organization's global perspective. *J Pain Symptom Manage.* 2002;24(2):91–96.

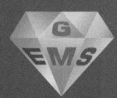

CHAPTER 10

Disaster Triage and Transporting Older Patients

LESSON OBJECTIVES

- Explain the planning process for the older adult population in disaster management.
- Identify special needs of the older adult population during a disaster.
- Demonstrate triage of older adult patients using the SWiFT triage tool in a disaster.
- Discuss evacuation and transportation of the older adult population during a disaster.

Introduction

A disaster can be defined as an event that causes a serious disruption in essential community services, resulting in crisis conditions. Disasters can be natural in origin or man-made. Disaster planners are facing many new challenges as the number and frequency of disasters increase at the same time as the older adult population grows in size. This demographic is more vulnerable to injury and death than the general population, and their mortality rate increases during and after a disaster.

Some natural disasters include wildfires, heat waves, tornados, hurricanes, tsunamis, and earthquakes. A United Nations report noted that older adults have disproportionately higher fatality rates during disasters worldwide. Scientists predict that with climate change, the severity and frequency of natural disasters will intensify.

Older adults are more vulnerable during a disaster due to many factors: They often have more chronic diseases that require medications or other daily management; may face mobility issues; may lack transportation or are unable to use transportation; may suffer more severe trauma due to age-related degeneration of the body, impaired vision and hearing, weakened immune systems, possible social isolation, inability to perform ADLs; and more (**FIGURE 10-1**).

Older adults, caregivers and family, and EMS practitioners all need to prepare for this special population in advance of a disaster, which can include stocking up on supplies, such as extra oxygen, medications, and first aid, and creating an evacuation plan.

Disaster Life Cycle

The life cycle of a disaster consists of five phases: prevention, mitigation, preparedness, response, and recovery (**TABLE 10-1**).

Phase 1: Prevention

Prevention is intended to ensure that human actions or natural phenomena do not result in disaster or emergency. This is a proactive phase in which potential hazards are identified and protection measures are implemented to reduce the impact of a disaster as much as possible. Ultimately, the goal is to prevent the disaster from occurring. For instance, installing smoke and carbon monoxide detectors in a long-term care facility is considered part of disaster prevention. Another example would be banning bonfires and backcountry travel during times of high risk for forest fires.

Critical Thinking Question

What is another example of a prevention phase task?

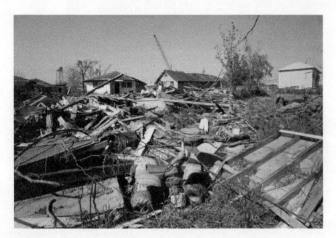

FIGURE 10-1 Hurricane damage can be devastating, especially for older adults, who may not be able to evacuate and become gravely injured; and, whose medical supplies can be destroyed or lost in the storm damage.

© Brian Nolan/Shutterstock

TABLE 10-1 Disaster Life Cycle

Phase	Actions
1. Prevention	Identify potential hazards and implement protection measures that could reduce the impact of a disaster
2. Mitigation	Actions taken to prevent or reduce the loss of life or the impact of a disaster, including risk assessments and disaster management strategies
3. Preparedness	Planning, training, and educational activities for people, organizations, and communities in the event a disaster cannot be mitigated
4. Response	Occurs after the disaster and includes short and long-term responses, including managing resources such as equipment, personnel, and supplies
5. Recovery	Beginning of restoration efforts to return to normal or a new normal of operations and activities; no set timeline

Phase 2: Mitigation

The mitigation phase includes actions to reduce loss of life and damage to property in advance of a disaster, including risk assessments and development of strategies to manage a disaster when it occurs. Disaster planning can occur at any level of government, from the local to federal level. Examples of actions taken during the mitigation phase could be implementing flood protection projects, changing building codes, or updating radio network systems for emergency responders.

Phase 3: Preparedness

Preparedness is a continuous process that includes planning, training, and educational activities for people, organizations, and communities to prepare for the effects of a disaster that cannot be mitigated. As part of your planning, be prepared for situations that don't fit in the "preparedness box" that is laid out in a plan or official guidelines. This may be more mental than supply-oriented, such as encountering an older adult with severe dementia who needs transport but doesn't want to leave.

Preparedness Pitfalls

Hurricane Harvey made landfall in Texas and Louisiana in 2017, causing disastrous flooding. The after-action report from Hurricane Harvey identified several issues that particularly affected older adults:

1. Red Cross nurses could not provide medical care at the shelters.
2. No functional needs assessments (SWiFT) were completed upon entry into the system.
3. Dialysis patients missed dialysis sessions.
4. Paratransit resources needed for the transport of the disabled were few and infrequent.

Check your local community protocols and resources to see if these measures are accounted for in case of a disaster.

Critical Thinking Questions

What issues might be identified after conducting a fire drill at a long-term care facility where most patients are unable to leave their beds and ambulate without assistance?

What solutions might be possible?

Phase 4: Response

The response phase occurs immediately after a disaster and can include short- and long-term responses. Measures are taken to reduce risks to life, property, and environment. Activities in this phase include coordinating resources such as equipment, personnel, and supplies; implementing response plans; removing hazards; conducting search and rescue operations; and directing the public as appropriate. Additional activities may include restoration of utilities, providing transport, and creating shelter options.

Communicating during a Disaster

Disasters exacerbate dementia, cognitive decline, and confusion in older adults, which could make treatment, evacuation, and transport more difficult. Effective communication is a critical tool in mitigating the effects of a disaster. Revisiting guidelines on how to work with patients with cognitive decline as part of your disaster planning is key.

Phase 5: Recovery

The recovery phase involves restorative efforts to return to the predisaster state or a new normal state of operations and activities. This phase could take weeks, months, or years. For instance, following the World Trade Center attacks, it took years for the community to return to a new normal of new buildings and heightened airport security, as well as other federal and local security measures and disaster response protocols. The recovery process involves prioritizing essential services such as food and water, utilities, transportation, and health care services. It can include rebuilding damaged structures to new code specifications to mitigate future risk or providing financial and mental health services for all community members affected by the disaster.

Critical Thinking Questions

What aspects of a disaster recovery are needed to assist older adult victims?

How does the management of older adults differ from that of younger victims?

Seniors without Families Team

The **Seniors Without Families Team (SWiFT)** is a triage tool that was developed in Houston after Hurricane Katrina. Postdisaster analysis showed that some older residents could not perform activities of daily living (ADLs) without assistance and did not know how to access or could not gain access to needed resources. The triage tool was designed to assess older adult residents in a shelter that had no caregivers available. This tool rapidly separates residents based on their independence performing ADLs. Once separated, each group can be assigned appropriate evacuation accommodations (**TABLE 10-2**).

SWiFT is only a triage tool. For it to be practical, a system must be in place to receive the triaged patients. Quick identification and transport of patients to appropriate facilities that can assist with ADLs and continued treatment of special needs could reduce mortality rates. Depending on the scale of the disaster, transport could involve long-term care facilities and hospitals in the same community or in nearby cities.

TABLE 10-2 SWiFT Triage	
SWiFT Level	**Ability Level**
Level 1	Unable to perform ADLs, including bathing, grooming, and eating. Requires transport to a long-term care facility as soon as possible.
Level 2	Unable to perform instrumental ADLs (IADLs) such as preparing meals, managing money, and using a phone. Requires assignment of a social care worker as soon as possible and accommodations that includes meals.
Level 3	Able to perform all ADLs and instrumental ADLs (IADLs). Requires connection with family, Red Cross, or other agency to assist with concerns, such as laundry services and transportation to medical appointments.

SWiFT Triage

SWiFT is an ideal tool for EMS as it rapidly assesses a group of geriatric patients and determines patient care needs as well as transport volume and modality required.

Critical Thinking Question

What tools are used in your region to identify the older adult population's needs in event of a disaster?

SWiFT and Disaster Transport of the Elderly

Evacuation of older adults is much more complicated than for other age groups, and it shares many of the same issues facing other disabled members of the community. Many older adult residents of long-term care facilities do not have family support available to them.

Independent older adults who do not require assistance with ADLs or IADLs can be evacuated in the same manner as other able-bodied age groups. The SWiFT tool used to determine appropriate disposition of evacuees can also be used to determine mode of transport.

SWiFT level 3 evacuees need assistance with transportation only. Suitable transportation for this group could include transit buses, tour buses, or school buses. This group will have a small amount of luggage and assistive equipment such as walkers, so extra space needs to be allocated, or a separate vehicle, such as a cargo truck or trailer, could be used.

SWiFT level 2 evacuees require accessible transport options, including paratransport services or accessible transit buses and school buses. Evacuees are typically transported in smaller groups, so luggage and specialized equipment they require may fit on the transport vehicle. Larger equipment, such as mobility scooters, may require trailer or cargo truck transport.

SWiFT level 1 evacuees vary in their transport needs. Modes of transport can range from accessible transport vehicles, to stretcher services, to critical care ambulances. Separate cargo transport vehicles may be needed for this group as well.

Consideration for patients requiring supplemental oxygen may mean provision of oxygen cylinders and availability of extra oxygen cylinders to replace those depleted during transport. Size and number of cylinders will dictate what type of vehicle can be used to meet safe transport requirements.

With so many transportation options, coordinating the evacuation of older adults is challenging. Disasters typically involve multiple agencies working together. As an EMS professional, you will need to be patient with the process, communicate clearly so your level of transport care is understood, and confirm the identity of your evacuee as well as the destination your evacuee has been assigned.

Once at your destination, provide a patient care report to the receiving caregiver and report to the facility transport coordinator that your transport has been completed. Providing confirmation that the evacuee has been relocated may mean contacting the person who originally assigned you the evacuation task.

Treatment and Transport

While isolated older adults remain one of the largest areas of concern during a disaster, there is an additional concern often not considered—older adults who are caregivers to others. You may only be expecting one person for transport, but upon arrival find a mixed household of the older adult's parent(s) who may be frail, perhaps a sibling or adult child with diminished mental capacity, and even grandchildren down to babies, as grandparents are often the default babysitters. Situations such as this should be part of your disaster planning and preparation.

CASE STUDY

You and your partner are working at an emergency response department as paramedics on an ambulance in a densely populated coastal tourist community. A category 3 hurricane eyewall is expected to pass 10 miles (15 km) south of your location. The storm is 300 miles (450 km) wide and has sustained winds of 128 mph (206 kph). There are reports that widespread flooding and severe structural damage are expected. There is also a risk of tornados in the area. Once the storm hits, you and your partner are expected to shelter in place at your station with one other EMS crew and ride out the storm. The department has stocked your station with 3 days of food and water provisions and other essential supplies.

QUESTIONS

- What "other essential supplies" would you stock at the station?
  - Clothes
  - Food
  - Water
  - Batteries
  - Medications
  - Spare glasses
- What type of damage would you expect from this type of storm?
  - Widespread flooding is a concern.
  - Heavy wind damage to structures with large debris fields can be anticipated.
  - Environmental concerns such as oil and septic spills, and flood waters increase the risk of contamination.
- What type of responses will there be once the storm has passed?
  - In addition to standard medical calls, the following types of specialized rescues could be needed:
    - Still water rescue
    - Swift water rescue
    - Entrapped patients
    - Confined space rescue

Approximately 12 hours before the hurricane will make landfall and prior to sheltering, you and your partner are dispatched to a local long-term care facility to assist with resident evacuations The facility is in a flood zone. You are advised by dispatch that you have been assigned to evacuate an unresponsive and ventilator-dependent 66-year-old patient.

QUESTIONS

- How will the weather conditions affect this response?
  - The weather conditions are deteriorating with rain and wind gusts up to 30 mph (48 kph). You and your partner decide it is still safe to respond despite the weather conditions. However, you should monitor weather updates to ensure the situation does not deteriorate or otherwise become more dangerous.
- What issues can occur when transporting a patient with a ventilator?
  - Dislodged tube
  - Obstruction
  - Equipment failure
  - Size of equipment to transport with patient
  - Possible need to ventilate patient with BVM during transport
- How will the patient's age affect your approach to prehospital patient care?
  - Given the age of the patient, using the GEMS Diamond as part of your assessment is appropriate.
- What equipment should you bring with you to your patient's side?
  - You decide to bring in the stretcher with rain cover, monitor, ventilator, airway kit, medicine kit, and suction based on the dispatch information.

You arrive at the front entrance of the long-term care home and are met at the door by a medical triage officer (MTO). The MTO hands you the patient's medical records and medications. While you don your PPE, the MTO directs you to transport the patient to a hospital 60 miles (96.6 km) away. As you make your way to the designated room, you note that the facility is chaotic, with patients being evacuated by multiple EMS agencies and stretcher services. Facility staff are collecting and providing equipment, documents, and

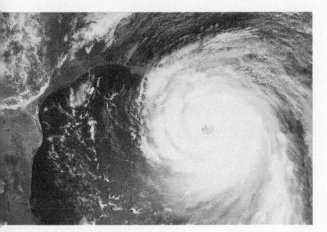

FIGURE 10-2

© Iavizzara/Shutterstock

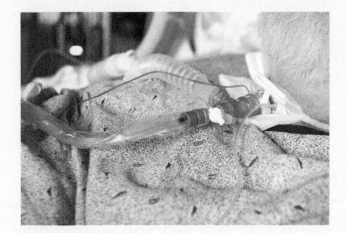

FIGURE 10-3

© Jana Shea/Shutterstock

medications to the MTO, who is coordinating the transportation and distributing the equipment and medications needed to the transport crews.

You arrive at your patient's room. You note that it is tidy, clean, has no hazards, and the temperature is warm. The patient is lying in bed and appears unresponsive and pale. He is intubated and ventilations are being provided mechanically. A facility nurse arrives to assist with the transfer to your stretcher. She confirms this is the correct patient, matching his medical bracelet with your documentation. She also confirms that the patient cannot perform any ADLs. His family lives in another part of the country and the facility is contacting them to advise them of the relocation.

You reference the patient's medical documents and note the patient has an advance directive that requests all medical care options are provided. You perform a primary survey and observe the following:

- X–No external bleeding apparent
- A–Airway is provided by a 7.5 mm endotracheal tube which is 21 cm at the lip and secured
- B–Mechanical ventilations by pressure SIMV (synchronized intermittent mechanical ventilations). Lungs are auscultated and wheezes are heard bilaterally.
- C–Radial pulses are strong, regular, and fast; skin is cool, dry, and pale
- D–GCS is 3T (E1, V1, M1), pupils are 5 mm, equal, and reactive
- E–No wounds, rash, or edema found

QUESTIONS

- Discuss any potential life threats identified in this case.
  - Potential life threats include displacement of the tube, obstruction, pneumothorax, and equipment failures that could lead to hypoxia and cardiac arrest.

- What would your initial treatment be?
  - Treatment should follow local guidelines and policy and be focused on supportive care and continuous airway and ventilatory status monitoring.

- What medication management should be performed, if any, en route to the receiving facility?
  - The patient is ventilator dependent. Medications could be needed to continue sedation for the long transport time.

- Where should the patient be transported?
  - This patient should be transported to the designated facility located out of town 60 miles (96.6 km).
  - Any diversion to another facility could delay care and further transport of additional patients needing to be removed from the hurricane's path.

Your partner assesses vital signs while you consult the facility staff and medical notes for the SAMPLER assessment. The patient is unresponsive and intubated, so you consult the documentation. Because this transport is due to a weather event, the chief complaint becomes the patient's condition that requires urgent transport to a distant hospital.

QUESTIONS

- What is the cardinal presentation and the chief complaint?
  - Cardinal presentation: Unresponsive
  - Chief complaint: Need for transport

- Are there any interventions required before assessment can continue?
  - No interventions are required, so you proceed with your assessment.

- What further assessments would you like to perform?
  - Using the GEMS approach, you and your partner assess vital signs, SAMPLER assessment, check the ventilator, perform an ECG and a physical head-to-toe examination.

Gather some history by using the SAMPLER mnemonic.

- S–Unresponsive, ventilator dependent
- A–Penicillin
- M–Staff state patient compliance with atorvastatin, lisinopril, irbesartan, aspirin, oxygen blended to 35%, levalbuterol, beclomethasone, insulin
- P–Hypertension, stroke, COPD, diabetes, and HF
- L–Received last feeding 3 hours ago via PEG tube
- E–Natural disaster is imminent and power for ventilator is not assured
- R–Age, stroke, diabetes, HF, resides in coastal region in flood zone

The vital signs are as follows:

- HR: 88
- SpO_2: 97% on 35% oxygen
- RR: 12 on ventilator
- BP: 136/94
- Temp: 97.6°F (36.4°C)
- $ETCO_2$: 41
- BGL: 86 mg/dl (4.8 mmol/l)

Ventilator settings are as follows:

- SIMV
- RR: 12
- Vt: 400
- PEEP: 5
- I:E ratio: 1:2

- ECG shows sinus tachycardia
- 12-lead ECG is unremarkable

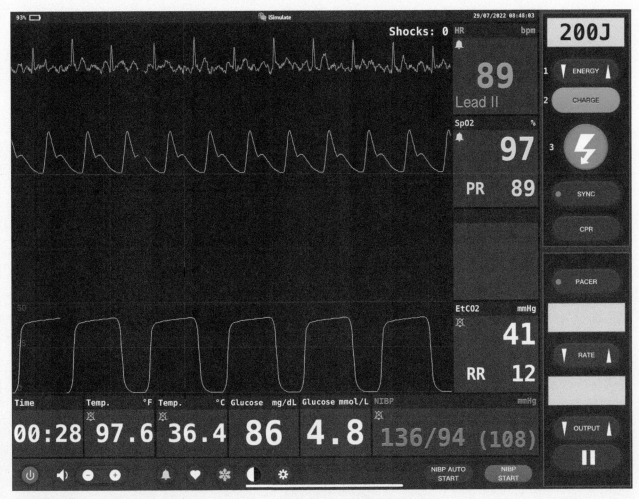

FIGURE 10-4

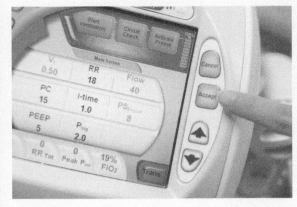

FIGURE 10-5

Head-to-toe assessment shows the following:

- HEENT
  - Head–Unremarkable
  - Eyes–PERRL
  - Ears–Unremarkable
  - Nose–Unremarkable
  - Throat–Unremarkable

- Heart and Lungs
  - Lung sounds: mild wheezing bilaterally.
  - Heart sounds are normal without murmur, rubs, or gallops.

- Neuro
  - Unresponsive

- Abdomen and Pelvis
  - Soft, nontender. Bowel sounds are normal.
  - Stage 2 pressure ulcer noted to the sacrum

- Upper Extremities
  - Unremarkable

- Lower Extremities
  - Unremarkable

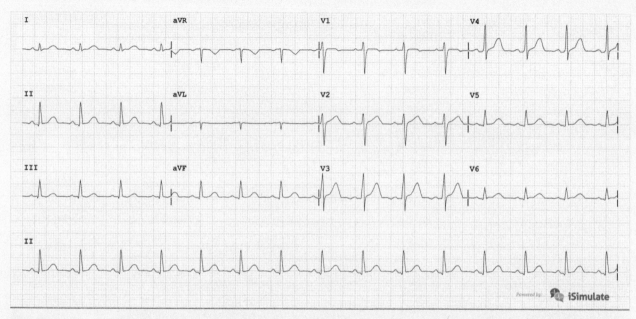

FIGURE 10-6

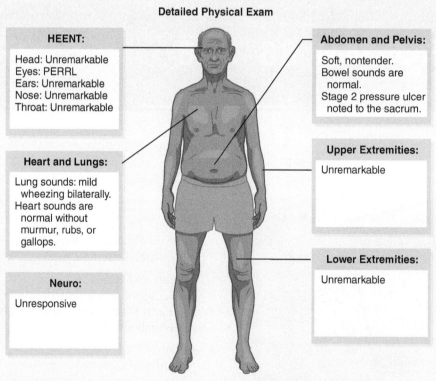

FIGURE 10-7

GEMS DIAMOND REVIEW

 Geriatric Assessment: The patient has more age-related changes than would be expected for a 66-year-old.

 Environmental Assessment: The room is clean and warm; the staff reports that the room is kept warmer for the patient's comfort. No odors noted.

 Medical Assessment: Facility staff report patient is compliant with medications and there have been no recent prescription changes.

 Social Assessment: The patient cannot accomplish ADLs by himself. He lives in a long-term care home, which provides all his support. His family lives a long distance away and rarely visits.

UESTIONS

- If you use your own ventilator, should you bring the patient's ventilator as well?
  - Discuss the importance of taking the patient's ventilator device with them to the receiving facility and how one could be secured.
  - Keep in mind that a facility may be reluctant to allow facility-owned equipment to leave with a patient due to the potential for lacking essential equipment needed during a disaster. Therefore, medical equipment should be included as part of the disaster planning.
  - Include options in the participant's region if they were unable to use the patient's ventilator for transport.
- What would you do if the ventilator stops functioning during transport?
  - Use of an EMS agency ventilator or BVM during transport are options.

reatment

- BLS
  - Position of comfort
  - Monitor vitals
  - Monitor airway and ventilations
  - Be prepared to ventilate with BVM
- ALS
  - BLS care
  - Monitor 12 lead
  - Be prepared for ET suction
- Critical care
  - BLS/ALS care

QUESTIONS

- How would you treat this patient according to your local protocol and scope of practice?
  - Ideally, this patient should be transported by an ALS or critical care crew.
  - Incident command should have a count of all responding agencies and their capabilities to ensure all patients are transported with the appropriate personnel.
  - Continuously monitor the patient's breathing and ventilatory status through $ETCO_2$, SPO_2, and auscultation.
  - Keep in mind the equipment should also be monitored and EMS practitioners should be prepared to control airway/ventilation in the event there is equipment failure.
- What are your goals for this patient?
  - The patient should be treated with supportive care.
  - Avoid aggressive treatment, as equipment could be limited during a disaster. For example, this patient does not need an IV and fluids. These could be saved for future patients. However, IV access should be maintained as the patient's condition could change quickly.
- How will you ensure the ventilator equipment is secure in the ambulance?
  - In the event of a quick maneuver, collision, or sudden braking, the ventilator equipment could serve as a hazard to the patient and provider and should be properly secured throughout transport.

You place the patient in a position of comfort onto the stretcher with the assistance of two facility staff. Once he has been moved, you confirm his endotracheal (ET) tube has not been displaced. Inadvertent misplacement of an ET tube, if unrecognized for only a brief period, may result in profound hypoxia. You confirm by verifying the

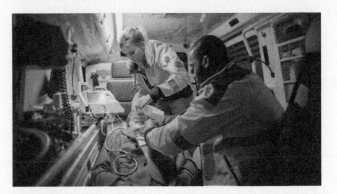

FIGURE 10-8

© Gorodenkoff/Shutterstock

depth at the lips, auscultating for bilateral breath sounds and presence of air sounds over the epigastrium, visualization of the chest rising and falling during ventilations, fogging in the ET tube on expiration, and capnography monitoring. Travel by ground is still considered safe so you transport the patient to the receiving hospital as planned. During transport, the ventilator low-pressure alarm sounds and shuts off 5 minutes from your destination. The ventilator is disconnected, and bag-valve mask ventilations are performed for the remainder of the trip. The patient is transferred to hospital care following your verbal and written reports. The patient was returned home to the long-term care facility after 5 days.

CASE STUDY WRAP-UP

Fifteen ambulances, two buses, and two trailers were used to evacuate 200 long-term care residents and their equipment. The ventilator patients were transferred first, followed by patients requiring supplemental oxygen. Patients were transported to various levels of care based on their needs, determined by the SWiFT tool, and capacity of receiving facilities. Patients were transported to other long-term care facilities, hospitals, hotel suites, and college dorms. Hotels and dorms were staffed by medical personnel including nurses and paramedics. Patients were transported with medication to last 5 days and personal belongings were limited.

CHAPTER WRAP-UP

Disaster management is critical to ensuring safety of the older adult population. All disasters require effective communication and teamwork. The SWiFT tool is a quick assessment to identify the geriatric community members who are the most in need of help.

REFERENCES

Baylor College of Medicine. Recommendations for best practices in the management of elderly disaster victims Harris County Hospital District. https://www.bcm.edu/pdf/bestpractices.pdf. Publication date unknown. Accessed April 2, 2021.

Dyer CB, Regev M, Burnett J, Festa N, Cloyd B. SWiFT: a rapid triage tool for vulnerable older adults in disaster situations. *Disaster Med Public Health Prep*. 2008;2(S1):S45–S50. doi:10.1097/dmp.0b013e3181647b81

FEMA. Livestock in disasters-Unit 4 emergency management in the United States. https://training.fema.gov/emiweb/downloads/is111_unit%204.pdf. Published October 31, 2013. Accessed May 3, 2021.

Gupta V, Lipsitz LA. Orthostatic hypotension in the elderly: diagnosis and treatment. *Am J Med*. 2007;120(10):841–847. doi:10.1016/j.amjmed.2007.02.023

Malik S, Lee DC, Doran KM, et al. Vulnerability of older adults in disasters: emergency department utilization by geriatric patients after Hurricane Sandy. *Disaster Med Public Health Prep*. 2017;12(2):184–193. doi:10.1017/dmp.2017.44

National Bureau of Economic Research. The long-run impacts of natural disasters on mortality and disease burden among U.S. elderly and disabled adults. https://www.nber.org/programs-projects/projects-and-centers/8065-long-run-impacts-natural-disasters-mortality-and-disease-burden-among-us-elderly-and-disabled?page=1&perPage=50. Published July 15, 2021.

National Council on Disability. The impact of Hurricanes Katrina and Rita on people with disabilities: a look back and remaining challenges. https://ncd.gov/publications/2006/Aug072006. Published August 3, 2006. Accessed May 13, 2021.

National Public Radio. Katrina took deadly toll on elderly. https://www.npr.org/templates/story/story.php?storyId=5242064#:~:text=More%20than%201%2C300%20people%20in. Published March 5, 2006. Accessed May 13, 2021.

National Weather Service. Historic July 12–15, 1995, heat wave. https://www.weather.gov/lot/1995_heatwave_anniversary. No date provided. Accessed on June 6, 2022.

Public Health Council of the Upper Valley. What is emergency preparedness—prevention mitigation preparedness response recovery. https://uvpublichealth.org/public-health-emergency-preparedness/prevention-mitigation-preparedness-response-recovery_03/. Publication date unknown. Accessed May 2, 2021.

Shultz JM, Galea S. Preparing for the Next Harvey, Irma, or Maria—addressing research gaps. *N Eng J Med*. 2017;377(19):1804–1806. doi:10.1056/nejmp1712854

St. Louis Missouri City Emergency Management Agency. Steps of emergency management. stlouis-mo.gov. https://www.stlouis-mo.gov/government/departments/public-safety/emergency-management/about/Steps-of-Emergency-Management.cfm#:~:text=Prevention%2C%20mitigation%2C%20preparedness%2C%20response. Published 2021. Accessed May 3, 2021.

Texas Health and Human Services. Hurricane Harvey response after-action report. https://www.tceq.texas.gov/assets/public/response/hurricanes/hurricane-harvey-after-action-review-report.pdf. Published May 30, 2018. Accessed April 6, 2021.

United Nations Department of Economic and Social Affairs. Current status of the social situation, well-being, participation in development and rights of older persons worldwide. https://www.un.org/esa/socdev/ageing/documents/publications/current-status-older-persons.pdf. New York, NY: United Nations; 2011.

Upton L, Kirsch TD, Harvey M, Hanfling D. Health care coalitions as response organizations: Houston after Hurricane Harvey. *Disaster Med Public Health Prep*. 2017;11(6):637–639. doi:10.1017/dmp.2017.141

CHAPTER 11

Left Ventricular Assist Devices

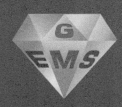

- Define a ventricular assist device (VAD) and describe the role it plays in treating heart failure.
- Review the basic equipment types, their settings, and operation.

- Describe the signs and symptoms of a patient with a malfunctioning LVAD.
- Identify how patients with LVADs are managed during a device malfunction.

Introduction

Heart function declines through the natural process of aging, which leads to a greater incidence of heart dysfunction in the geriatric population (**FIGURE 11-1**). Much research has gone into the management of patients with heart dysfunction and failure. Given the mechanics of the heart, research has not been limited to medical and surgical interventions. A variety of new equipment has been invented that can lessen the effect of heart failure. Ventricular assist devices (VADs) are not artificial hearts, but they can temporarily support a failing heart, provide improved quality of life, and bridge the patient to a more permanent solution. They are mechanical pumps used to improve blood flow in people with weakened hearts.

The types of VADs are classified as left ventricular assist device (LVAD), right ventricular assist device (RVAD), and biventricular assist device (BiVAD), and further subtypes include pulsatile flow devices and continuous flow devices. This chapter focuses on LVADs, as they are the ones most likely to be encountered by EMS practitioners, but all three types are similar in their basic function.

Physiology of Heart Failure

The gradual failure of the largest functional unit of the heart, the left ventricle, leads to decreasing ability to pump blood from the pulmonary veins to the aorta and the body (**FIGURE 11-2**). This failure leads to blood backing up in the pulmonary system, which increases the blood pressure within the pulmonary system. The increased pressure within the blood vessels forces fluid out of the bloodstream, through the capillary walls, and into the alveolar space in the lungs. The condition of circulatory fluid displacing air within the alveoli is called **pulmonary edema**.

When the right ventricle of the heart fails, it becomes unable to pump blood from the inferior vena cava and the superior vena cava to the pulmonary trunk and the lungs. This causes blood to back up into the systemic vasculature. The superior vena cava drains blood from the upper body so back up of blood in this vasculature will cause the jugular veins to engorge and visibly distend. The inferior vena cava receives blood from the hepatic system, veins draining the digestive system, and tissues of the lower body.

Similar to left ventricular failure, increasing pressure within the vasculature due to blood backing up forces fluid within the bloodstream to be forced through the capillary walls. This displaced fluid presents as hepatomegaly, or enlarged liver, in the hepatic system and edema, or tissue swelling, in the tissues of the lower body. Because of the effects of gravity, displaced fluid from the capillaries in the lower body will settle to the lowest body parts. Typically, this edema is seen in the lower legs and is called **peripheral edema**.

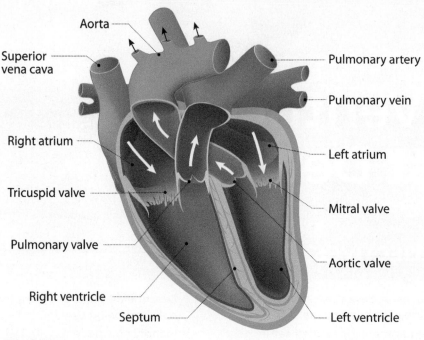

FIGURE 11-1 Heart anatomy.

© Designua/Shutterstock

Chronic failure of the heart is known as heart failure (HF; formerly congestive heart failure; **TABLE 11-1**). Once the diagnosis of HF is made, there are many therapies available for managing it, including medication, surgery, and invasive devices such as implanted cardioverter defibrillators and VADs.

There are approximately 400,000 new cases of HF in the United States every year, and roughly 2 million Americans are living with the disorder.

Left Ventricular Assist Device

Of the three types of VADs, the LVAD is the most common (**FIGURE 11-3**). The number of patients with LVADs is increasing every year, as is the EMS exposure to this type of patient. Understanding how the device works,

TABLE 11-1 Causes of Heart Failure

Disorder	Pathology
Coronary artery disease	Narrowing of the artery lumen due to build-up of plaque leads to decreased blood supply to the heart muscle over time; may cause an acute myocardial infarction (AMI).
Previous AMIs	Infarcted muscle tissue is dead muscle tissue that does not contract or transmit a depolarizing stimulus.
Chronic uncontrolled hypertension	The heart must work harder to pump blood when it is under pressure. This causes the left ventricle to become thicker, stiffer, and less efficient.
Abnormal heart valves	Valves do not fully open or close as they should, so the heart's pumping is inefficient due to increased resistance during systole or backflow during diastole.
Heart muscle diseases and disorders	Inflammation or genetic enlargement will decrease efficiency of cardiac muscle contraction and pumping.

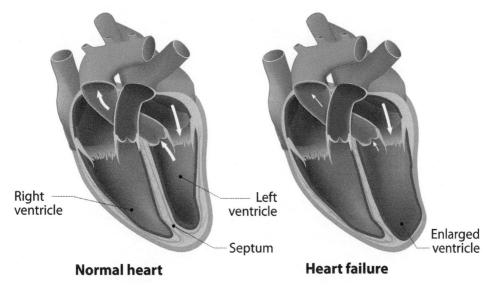

Right ventricle

Left ventricle

Septum

Normal heart

Enlarged ventricle

Heart failure

FIGURE 11-2 Heart failure.
© Designua/Shutterstock

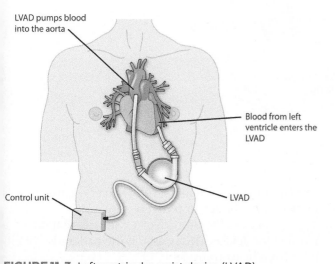

LVAD pumps blood into the aorta

Blood from left ventricle enters the LVAD

Control unit

LVAD

FIGURE 11-3 Left ventricular assist device (LVAD).
© Blamb/Shutterstock

the problems you may encounter with it, and how to manage a patient with an LVAD is necessary.

LVAD Function

An LVAD takes over the work of a weakened and ineffective left ventricle. It is surgically attached to the left ventricle and the aorta. Blood is drawn from the left ventricle apex and pumped into the ascending aorta. Depending on the type of LVAD, blood is circulated using a pulsatile pump or a continuous flow pump. The components of an LVAD are described in **TABLE 11-2**.

The LVAD pulsatile pump functions much like the left ventricle with a pumping, or systolic, phase, and a

pause, or diastolic, phase (**FIGURE 11-4**). Blood enters a collapsible chamber that is squeezed at a set rate to force the blood into systemic circulation. You may be able to palpate a pulse and assess a blood pressure if the heart is strong enough. Auscultation at the heart apex will reveal the sound of the chamber collapsing. This type of LVAD was an early design and is not placed as often as continuous flow devices.

The LVAD continuous flow pump propels blood forward with a spinning impeller (**FIGURE 11-5**). Patients with this type of device may have a weak, irregular, or nonpalpable pulse, depending on the degree of underlying heart failure. Assess for good working status by auscultating a continuous humming sound at the heart apex. Blood flow is determined by the revolving speed of the impeller, which is normally 2,000 to 10,000 revolutions per minute. The blood flow rate is determined and set by the VAD clinical team and typically cannot be manipulated outside the hospital. Obtaining a manual blood pressure is difficult to impossible. Doppler ultrasound can be used to assess blood pressure.

When being used, the patient's diastolic pressure will be increased and the pulse pressure decreased since blood flow will be occurring during the diastole

No Pulse?

Because the continuous flow type of LVAD is continuously pumping blood, the pulse pressure is so reduced that it may not be palpable at the carotid or radial pulse points.

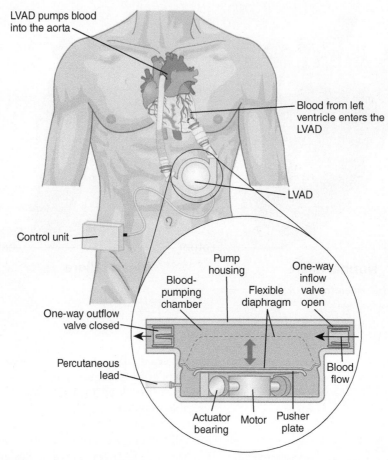

LVAD pumps blood into the aorta

Blood from left ventricle enters the LVAD

LVAD

Control unit

Pump housing

Blood-pumping chamber

One-way inflow valve open

Flexible diaphragm

One-way outflow valve closed

Blood flow

Percutaneous lead

Actuator bearing

Motor

Pusher plate

FIGURE 11-4 Pulsatile-flow LVAD.

© Jones & Bartlett Learning

Critical Thinking Question

What would happen if you administered nitroglycerin to an LVAD patient complaining of chest pain?

period. Because the pump can only move the blood it receives, LVAD patients are very **preload** dependent.

Indications for LVAD Use

The most common reason for receiving an LVAD is to bridge the patient to heart transplant. The LVAD is used to provide circulatory support to allow for rehabilitation from severe HF while waiting for a donor organ. This is referred to as bridge to transplant.

It may also be used as a temporary measure to provide circulatory support in patients with HF who have undergone a cardiac procedure and require improved

cardiac function to make a full recovery. This usage is referred to as bridge to recovery.

Destination therapy involves the placement of a permanent device. This is used if the patient is not eligible for a heart transplant.

Bridge to candidacy or bridge to decision is a short-term use of an LVAD on a patient presenting with end-organ dysfunction due to HF. Use of the LVAD may improve the patient's health status enough to become eligible for a heart transplant.

Contraindications for LVAD Use

Although LVAD use can be lifesaving, there are many contraindications to its use (**TABLE 11-3**).

Patients must be compliant with medications and the directions for care and use of an LVAD. Because LVAD malfunction will result in unconsciousness, caregivers must also receive extensive training on device operation, maintenance, and response required for each alarm.

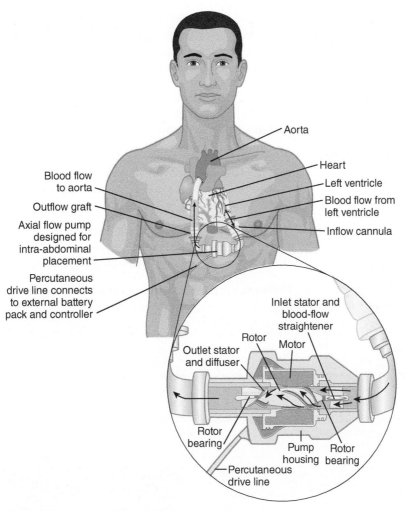

FIGURE 11-5 Continuous flow LVAD.
© Jones & Bartlett Learning

TABLE 11-2 LVAD Components	
Inflow cannula	A tube attached to the inferior left ventricle that leads to the pumping mechanism and allows blood flow through
Outflow conduit	A tube attached to the pump that leads to the aorta and allows blood to pass through
Pump	Implanted in the upper abdomen and pumps blood received from the left ventricle into the aorta
Driveline	Passed through the abdominal wall and connects to an external controller to allow for power to run the pump and wiring to allow for monitoring pump function; also referred to as the percutaneous lead
Controller	Worn by the patient externally and sounds alarm warnings for low power or pump dysfunction
Power source	Provided by direct connection to alternating current (AC) power or by batteries worn externally by the patient

TABLE 11-3 Contraindications for LVAD Use

Right ventricular dysfunction	The LVAD requires preload into the left ventricle to work properly. An efficient right ventricle is needed to provide this.
Neurologic compromise caused by acute cardiogenic shock	LVAD placement will increase morbidity and decrease quality of life of patients with severe brain injury postcardiac arrest or after a period of cerebral hypoperfusion.
Noncardiac life-threatening illness	Patients with life-threatening illness will have increased morbidity and decreased quality of life following LVAD placement. This includes pulmonary, hepatic, renal, or neurologic disorders, and advanced metastatic cancer.
Bleeding disorder	Patients require anticoagulation following LVAD placement. Patients with active bleeding, thrombocytopenia, or heparin-induced thrombocytopenia would not be able to tolerate the treatment.
Hypertrophic cardiomyopathy or large ventricular septal defect	Prevents proper placement and functioning of an LVAD.
Body surface area of 13 to 16 square feet (1.2 to 1.5 m²) or less	Patient is too small for proper placement and functioning of LVAD.
Patient and caregiver compliance	Compliance with medications and equipment maintenance is critical for successful use.

Copyright © 2024 National Association of Emergency Medical Technicians (NAEMT).

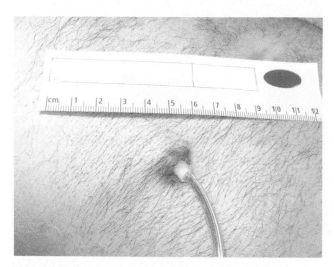

FIGURE 11-6 LVAD driveline infection at exit point.
© John-Fs-Pic/Shutterstock

Complications

Potential complications include infection (**FIGURE 11-6**), bleeding, embolic stroke or transient ischemic attack, hemolysis, arrythmias, volume overload, dehydration, hypertension, hypotension, cardiac tamponade, recurrence of HF, new right ventricular heart failure, and aortic insufficiency.

Look for Infection

The most common complication of LVAD placement is infection.

Treatment

Most LVAD devices have a tag located on the controller, which is worn on the waist (**FIGURE 11-7**). The tag includes pertinent information like the type of implanted device, the institution that implanted it, and an emergency number to contact for assistance. The tag will be a specific color to correspond with an EMS field guide that can be accessed at the MyLVAD website at www.mylvad.com/ems. The field guide provides necessary information for EMS practitioners to manage the patient's device. Caregivers (if present) are well trained in troubleshooting techniques and emergency care and are therefore excellent resources. Troubleshooting a device when alarms are sounding should not delay transport.

It is important to identify whether the patient's device is the continuous flow type or pulsatile type. Patients with continuous flow pumps could have an unreliable pulse oximetry reading due to low pulse

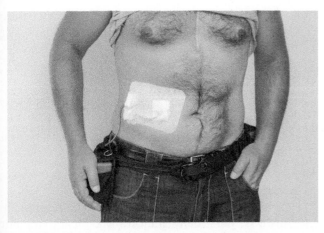

FIGURE 11-7 Most devices have a tag located on the controller around the waist, as shown here. The tag includes all required information about the device, an emergency phone number to contact for assistance, and will be a specific color to correspond with an EMS Field Guide that can be found using the MyLVAD website.

© John-Fs-Pic/Shutterstock

pressure generated by the device. Pulsatile pumps should not have any effect on the pulse pressure or blood pressure.

Continuously More Common

Continuous flow LVADs are more common than pulsatile LVADs.

Patients presenting with stroke symptoms should be transported to a stroke center capable of managing patients with LVADs. Airway interventions, ventilatory support, and intravenous therapy must be managed just as for patients without LVADs. Arrhythmias are managed only if they are causing symptoms.

A 12-lead ECG can provide critical information regarding the patient's status. However, while an LVAD does not interfere with ECG interpretation, defibrillation pads, or therapy electrodes should not be placed on top of the device, meaning placement will need to be in the anterior-posterior position. There are no contraindications to the administration of antiarrhythmics, but vasopressors should be used with caution; because they increase afterload, the pump may not be able to compensate. Transport the patient to the most appropriate facility along with a family member or caregiver (if available) who is familiar with the device.

CASE STUDY

You and your partner are working for an emergency ambulance service in a suburban area. You are dispatched to a house for a 68-year-old male complaining of shortness of breath. It is a fall morning with an air temperature of 48°F (8.9°C).

QUESTIONS

- What is on your differential diagnosis list?
  - You and your partner discuss the potential differential diagnosis as you respond. The complaint of shortness of breath is nonspecific, so many body systems can be involved. Differential diagnosis includes the following:
    - Pneumonia
    - Pulmonary embolism (PE)
    - Pneumothorax
    - AMI
    - COVID-19
    - Anxiety
    - Allergies
    - COPD/HF exacerbation
    - Toxic inhalation
    - Asthma
    - Sepsis

- How does the patient's age affect your assessment approach?
  - You decide that you will include the GEMS approach to your assessment due to the patient's age.

- What equipment should you bring with you to your patient's side?
  - You decide to bring the stretcher, oxygen, med kit, defibrillator, and airway kit.

You arrive at the patient's house. It appears safe and you put on your routine personal protective equipment (PPE), go to the front door, and are met by the patient's neighbor. He leads you into the kitchen where the patient is sitting in a chair by the table. The residence is untidy, but no significant obstacles are present. The garbage bin contains empty alcohol bottles and there is an alcohol odor in the air. The house is warm and well lit.

The neighbor advises you that the patient lives alone. He had not seen the patient out in his yard for a couple days, so he dropped in and found him in this condition. He tells you that the patient is a heavy drinker and "has heart problems." He is divorced and has no children. A home health nurse checks on him three times a week.

Your general impression is that the patient is alert, his work of breathing is increased, and his skin is flushed. He smells of alcohol and appears to be intoxicated. The scene appears safe, and you deem your PPE is appropriate, so you approach the patient. You note he is wearing two packs at his side and a controller around his waist that appears to be an LVAD. You note redness around the drive line that is tunneled in the abdomen.

You perform a primary survey and find the following:

- X–No hemorrhage noted.
- A–Patent airway.
- B–Breathing is rapid and labored; lungs are auscultated and are clear bilaterally; SpO$_2$ 88% room air.
- C–Radial pulses are absent; skin is warm and clammy.
- D–GCS is 14 (E4, V4, M6), pupils are 5, equal, and sluggish.

- E–No wounds, rash, or edema found; patient wearing LVAD battery and controller with inflammation a the LVAD percutaneous lead site.

QUESTIONS

- What is the cardinal presentation and the chie complaint?
  - Cardinal presentation: Respiratory distress and altered mental status
  - Chief complaint: Difficulty breathing

- Are any life threats present?
  - This patient is exhibiting signs of respiratory distress, potentially indicating a life threat, bu more assessment is needed.

- Are any interventions required before assessmen can continue?
  - You immediately provide high-flow oxygen by nonrebreather mask.

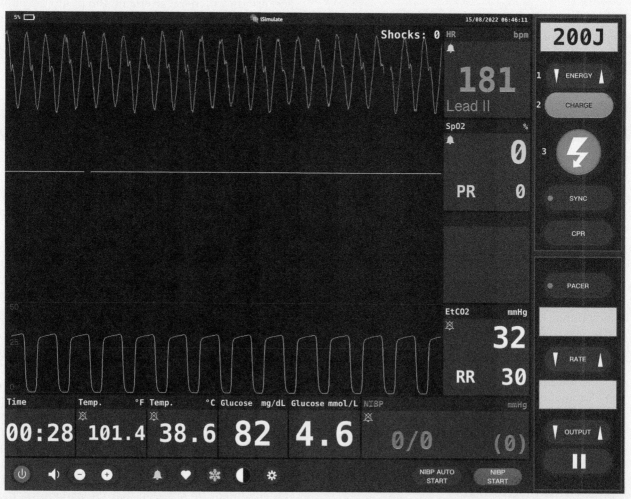

FIGURE 11-8

- Does this patient require immediate transport, or can you remain on scene and continue your assessment?
  - Though immediate transport is not required, you and your partner discuss transport decisions. This patient should be transported to the closest, most appropriate facility capable of managing VADs.

After oxygen has been provided, your partner assesses vital signs while you consult the patient and medical records at his home used by the home health nurse for the OPQRST of this shortness of breath and SAMPLER assessments.

- O–Sudden
- P–Improves when sitting upright, worsens when supine
- Q–Air hunger
- R–None
- S–10/10
- T–15 minutes
- S–Shortness of breath, redness around the percutaneous lead/skin border
- A–NKA
- M–Compliant with labetalol, valsartan, rivaroxaban, eplerenone, potassium
- P–End-stage heart failure, AMIs, hypertension, continuous flow LVAD in situ
- L–A few bites of a sandwich an hour ago
- E–Was walking in the house when shortness of breath started, feeling unwell for 2 days
- R–Age, severe heart disease, LVAD, hypertension

Vital Signs

- HR: Is tachycardic
- SpO$_2$: 88% with high-flow oxygen by nonrebreather mask
- RR: 28
- BP: 68/Doppler
- Temp: 101.4°F (38.2°C)
- ETCO$_2$: 32 mm Hg
- BGL: 81 mg/dl (4.6 mmol/l)

A 12-lead ECG shows ventricular tachycardia.

You know that SpO$_2$ is not reliable with LVAD and no pulsatile flow. The patient's ETCO$_2$ is low, which could be in part due to low blood pressure, but there could be other causes. V-tach is common in patients with VAD, and blood flow is not determined by patient's intrinsic heart rate but by the VAD. V-tach should not affect the function of the VAD and should not be cardioverted unless directed to do so by the VAD coordinator. You are concerned, as the patient's respiration, temperature, and blood pressure are consistent with criteria for sepsis. The redness around the LVAD driveline could indicate an infection and possible sepsis.

A physical head-to-toe assessment is performed and you note that his abdomen is soft and tender to touch in all quadrants. There are no other new findings.

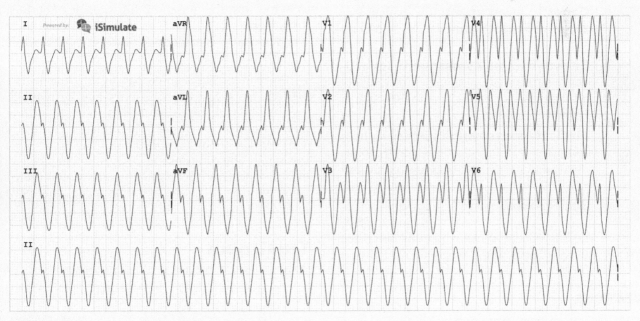

FIGURE 11-9

Detailed Physical Exam

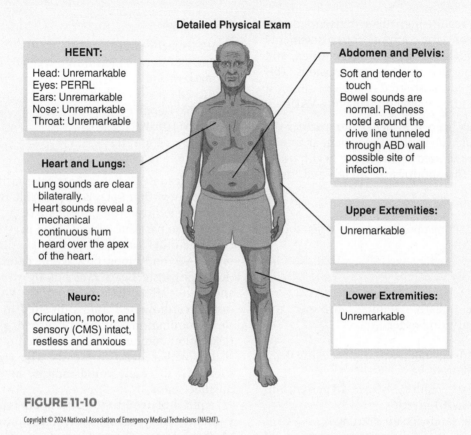

HEENT:

Head: Unremarkable
Eyes: PERRL
Ears: Unremarkable
Nose: Unremarkable
Throat: Unremarkable

Heart and Lungs:

Lung sounds are clear bilaterally.
Heart sounds reveal a mechanical continuous hum heard over the apex of the heart.

Neuro:

Circulation, motor, and sensory (CMS) intact, restless and anxious

Abdomen and Pelvis:

Soft and tender to touch
Bowel sounds are normal. Redness noted around the drive line tunneled through ABD wall possible site of infection.

Upper Extremities:

Unremarkable

Lower Extremities:

Unremarkable

FIGURE 11-10

GEMS DIAMOND REVIEW

 Geriatric Assessment: The patient has age-related changes expected for a 68-year-old, plus advanced heart disease.

 Environmental Assessment: His residence appears safe, although untidy. Empty alcohol containers in kitchen with odor of alcohol.

 Medical Assessment: Patient states he is compliant with medications and appointments and there have been no recent prescription changes; LVAD is in place.

 Social Assessment: The patient is independent and divorced, with no children; he has a health nurse who visits him three times a week and a neighbor who checks on him.

QUESTIONS

- Why is his oxygen saturation remaining so low despite 100% oxygen?
  - Pulse oximetry is unreliable in patients with continuous flow LVADs due to the low pulse pressure generated.

- Why was the onset of his shortness of breath sudden?
  - Sudden onset of shortness of breath could be a failure of the LVAD, though there may be other causes.

The patient has a to-go bag by his side with cables, chargers, and extra batteries and he requests it be brought with him. His medical records include a phone number for his VAD coordinator. You call the VAD coordinator and report the situation and your assessments. She confirms the LVAD is functioning based on the continuous hum you auscultated and the controller settings, including the pump speed, flow, power, and remaining battery life.

Treatment

- BLS
  - Call VAD coordinator and give a report of the patient's condition.
    - Monitor airway.
    - Administer humidified oxygen.
    - Consider ventilatory assistance.
    - Administer acetaminophen for fever.
  - Place in position of comfort.

- ALS
  - BLS care
  - Consult with VAD coordinator:
    - Start an IV and give fluid bolus.
    - Consider synchronized cardioversion.
- Critical care
  - BLS/ALS care.
  - Monitor for signs of respiratory failure and need for rapid sequence intubation (RSI).
  - Administer antibiotics.

QUESTIONS

- What does your differential diagnosis list include now?
  - VAD malfunction
  - Pneumonia
  - AMI
  - COVID-19
  - COPD/HF exacerbation
  - Sepsis
- How should you manage the V-tach?
  - In patients with VADs, dysrhythmias should only be managed if they are symptomatic; in this case, auscultation revealed a continuous hum, which suggests that the LVAD is functioning properly, and the patient's symptoms are not likely to be related to the V-tach. Also, you should always check with the VAD coordinator before initiating care related to the LVAD.
- Should you treat the blood pressure?
  - Given that VADs are preload-dependent, vasopressors should be used very cautiously. Fluid could be considered in cases of hypovolemia, but

fluid overload is a risk in all patients with heart failure. Again, check with the VAD coordinator for instructions.

- What are your goals for this patient?
  - Treat patient with supportive care.
  - Be prepared for rapid deterioration.
  - Identify promptly respiratory distress, failure, and/or arrest and intervene if escalation of therapy is required.
- Would bronchodilators work for this patient?
  - There is no evidence for need of a bronchodilator.
  - There is no wheezing, and the $ETCO_2$ waveform does not demonstrate loss of alveolar plateau (shark fin).
- What is the best transportation destination for this patient?
  - The patient should be transported to the closest appropriate facility with VAD capabilities.

The VAD coordinator does not recommend synchronized cardioversion to correct the V-tach since the LVAD is functioning normally. The VAD coordinator also recommends immediate transport since there has been no clinical improvement despite humidified oxygen therapy. Intravenous access can be established and a fluid bolus is administered. You begin rapid transport of the patient to the regional hospital that has VAD capabilities at the VAD coordinator's direction, even though it is not the closest hospital. You continuously monitor the patient during transport and prepare to provide positive-pressure ventilations and RSI. There is evidence the patient is getting worse, as SpO_2 does not rise, and the patient appears more agitated and restless. The $ETCO_2$ remains low. There are no further changes during transport.

CASE STUDY WRAP-UP

On arrival at the hospital, oxygen therapy is continued and blood samples are collected for lab evaluation. Lab results indicate a bacterial infection is present and a broad-spectrum antibiotic is administered. The diagnosis is gradual onset of confusion, fever, and tachypnea due to sepsis. Sepsis can occur in patients who wear a VAD for extended periods of time.

The patient is transferred to the VAD center where the device was implanted. He was discharged 7 days later to a nursing/rehab facility for a 30-day rehab plan. Recommendations are made for his admission to a long-term care facility.

CHAPTER WRAP-UP

VADs are preload dependent. Any medications that decrease preload or any cause for hypotension can severely compromise the effectiveness of the LVAD.

Preload can be corrected with a fluid bolus or VAD coordinator–directed changing of the settings on the controller.

Thrombosis and sepsis are common complications associated with those wearing VADs. Look for signs of infection in the tunneled drive line.

Check an ECG for all patients with VADs, as V-tach can be a common rhythm patients could be in. If the patient is in V-fib or V-tach, electrical therapy should be at the recommendation of the VAD coordinator only. Contact the closest VAD coordinator or cardiac transplant center as soon as possible. All VAD wearers have VAD coordinators they can contact 24/7 and they should be your go-to person.

REFERENCES

American Heart Association. Causes of Heart Failure. Last reviewed May 31, 2017. Accessed May 25, 2021. https://www.heart.org/en/health-topics/heart-failure/causes-and-risks-for-heart-failure/causes-of-heart-failure

Brito D, Cepeda B. Heart Failure, Congestive (CHF). Updated September 24, 2021. Accessed May 25, 2021. https://www.ncbi.nlm.nih.gov/books/NBK430873/

Modi K, Pannu AK, Modi RJ, et al. Utilization of left ventricular assist device for congestive heart failure: inputs on demographic and hospital characterization from nationwide inpatient sample. *Cureus*. Published online July 1, 2021. doi:10.7759/cureus.16094

Vaidya Y, Riaz S, Dhamoon AS. Left Ventricular Assist Devices (LVAD). Updated July 1, 2021. Accessed May 26, 2021. https://www.ncbi.nlm.nih.gov/books/NBK499841/

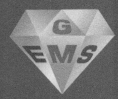

CHAPTER 12

Skin Disorders

LESSON OBJECTIVES

- Discuss the epidemiology, pathophysiology, assessment, intervention, and transport of older patients with skin disorders.

- Identify the stages of pressure ulcers.
- Discuss the prevention and management of skin disorders.

Introduction

Skin is the body's number one defense mechanism against infection. Therefore, breakdown of the skin due to aging puts the older person at greater risk of infection, compounded by higher risk due to a weakened immune system. More than 27 million people visit dermatologists annually and most of these patients are older than 65 years. The incidence of dermatologic disorders increases each year as the population of older adults continues to grow.

Skin Cancer

More than 5 million annual visits to a dermatologist involve new skin cancers.

Skin Anatomy and Aging

There are three major layers of skin and each is affected by aging (**FIGURE 12-1**).

1. The epidermis serves as the protective outer layer, which contains pores, pigment, and ducts. This layer is constantly shedding upper dead cells. New cells are constantly regenerated to replace those dead cells, but this slows down with aging. Cell regeneration is 70% slower for people in their 70s than when they were in their 20s.

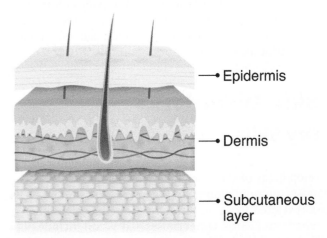

FIGURE 12-1 Three main layers of the skin.
© solar22/Shutterstock

The dermal-epidermal junction transfers nutrients from the dermis to the epidermal layer. This layer flattens with age so there is less nutrient transfer. As a result, the epidermal layer becomes more fragile, and the older adult becomes more prone to skin tears, bruising, and blisters. Wound healing time is also increased.

2. The dermis is the middle layer; it helps protect against trauma and is involved with thermoregulation. There is less blood flow as a person ages, so the skin appears pale and feels cooler. The reduced blood flow also reduces the thermoregulation function of the skin, including sweat production.

151

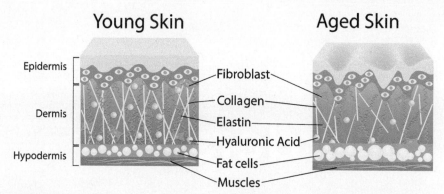

FIGURE 12-2 Changes in the three layers of the skin due to the aging process.
© Sofia Bessarab/Shutterstock

Altered protein levels and loss of oil glands associated with aging means that skin becomes rough, dry, flaky, and itchy. Cutaneous nerve endings that sense pain, pressure, and temperature decrease so there is a greater risk of severe injury due to lack of sensation in older adults.

3. The subcutaneous layer (hypodermis) is the innermost layer of the skin. This layer also provides protection from trauma and provides an insulating barrier to limit heat loss. The subcutaneous layer also becomes thinner with age, which contributes to wrinkle formation (**FIGURE 12-2**).

Skin Disorders

Dry Skin

Due to normal age-related changes, people will develop areas of skin that appear rough and scaly. This is most commonly found on the lower arms and legs. Dry skin related to aging is due to the reduced number of sebaceous glands. Other causes of dry skin include poor hydration, environmental dry air, excessive sun exposure, stress, smoking, health disorders such as diabetes or kidney disease, and adverse medication effect.

Thinning and dry skin reduces the skin's resistance to microorganisms. Thus, preventing dry skin can reduce the incidence of skin tears and infections. Preventative steps include the use of moisturizers and lotions daily, washing with mild soap, reducing the frequency of baths or showers, bathing with warm water instead of hot, and humidifying dry environments.

Skin Tears and Bruising

Skin tears are due to loss of elasticity in the dermal skin layer plus a thinner and weaker epidermal skin layer. Minor force on the skin, such as too firm a grip while lifting a patient's arm, can cause tearing and bruising

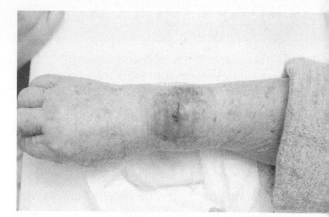

FIGURE 12-3 Reduced elasticity, weakened blood vessels, diminished subcutaneous fat, and some medications cause older skin to bruise very easily.
© BBbirdZ/Shutterstock

(**FIGURE 12-3**). Weakened vessels in the subcutaneous and dermal layers increase the likelihood of bleeding into the skin layers, causing the skin to easily bruise.

Common factors associated with skin tears and bruising in older adults include the following:

- Sensory loss
- Deficient nutrition
- Dehydration
- Age greater than 70 years
- Poor skin care

Treatment for a skin tear is much the same as for a laceration. Avoid using tape or adhesive bandages as their removal will likely result in more skin tears.

Critical Thinking Question

How should you secure an intravenous line on a patient over the age of 70?

oller gauze is preferred to tape. Patients on anticoagulant medications may require firm direct pressure and additional bandaging.

kin Cancer

kin cancer predominantly occurs in patients 65 years nd older. Skin cancers can be categorized into groups ch as cutaneous melanoma (CM) and nonmelanoma in cancer (NMSC). CM is caused by multiple factors nd its frequency is increasing more rapidly than any her form of cancer. The median age of diagnosis is years. The primary environmental cause is intermitnt and intense exposure to ultraviolet light. In other ords, a history of repeated sunburns is associated ith a high risk. There is also increased risk if there is a mily history of developing CM.

Melanoma Flip-Flop

Cutaneous melanoma affects more women at a younger age than men; however, more men are affected than women after age 55.

NMSC is the most common cancer affecting those with lighter skin tones. Of all types of skin cancers, 80% are NMSC (**FIGURE 12-4**). This includes basal cell carcinoma, accounting for 70%, and cutaneous squamous cell carcinoma. In 2012, approximately 3.3 million Americans were treated for NMSC. This represents a 35% increase in cases over the previous 6-year period. However, reporting of NMSC is largely underestimated because these tumors are not recorded in the national cancer registries. As with CM, NMSC is caused by intermittent exposure to ultraviolet light and genetics. Studies have shown that, despite an increasing incidence of NMSC, there is a stable or decreasing mortality rate associated with it. Prehospital intervention is typically sought due to adverse medication effect or infection of a surgical site. If wound care is needed, avoid the use of tape as it may further damage the skin.

Pressure Ulcers

Pressure ulcers are areas of tissue death (necrosis) caused by decreased tissue perfusion as a result of prolonged direct pressure. Areas prone to pressure ulcers are sites where there is a thin layer of tissue above a bony prominence in contact with a hard surface. For

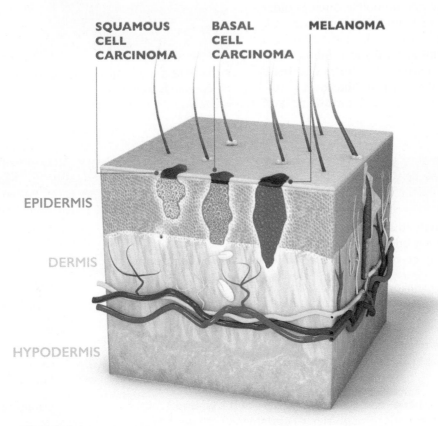

FIGURE 12-4 Types of skin cancer.

instance, tissues covering the sacrum will be compressed when a person is laying supine. Other common sites include the greater trochanter and the ischial tuberosity at the hip, the calcaneus at the heel, the scapula at the shoulder, and the fibular head at the knee. Ninety-five percent of pressure ulcers occur in the lower part of the body. The time it takes for a pressure ulcer to form depends on the strength of the skin and presence of moisture and can range from 1 to 24 hours.

A Wound by Any Other Name

Pressure ulcers are also known as decubitus ulcers, bed sores, or pressure sores.

Pressure ulcers can also be caused by friction or shearing forces that can occur when sliding on a firm surface. Friction and shearing forces reduce blood flow by stretching the subcutaneous tissue. Moisture, such as caused by urinary incontinence, can weaken the skin, making it more susceptible to injury from pressure or friction.

Approximately 1.5 million patients in the United States receive treatment annually for pressure ulcers. Patients who are inactive and immobile, such as older adults, those with spine or brain injury, or those with neuromuscular disorder, are at risk of developing a pressure ulcer. Malnutrition, fecal incontinence, urinary incontinence, and neuropathies further increase the risk. Pressure ulcers that occur on the coccyx, buttocks, or genital area may be exposed to urine or fecal

matter, particularly in bed-bound patients who wear incontinence briefs. The risk of infection leading to sepsis is higher in these patients (**FIGURE 12-5**).

Stages of Pressure Ulcers

TABLE 12-1 explains the four stages of pressure ulcer presentation and **FIGURE 12-6** provides an illustration of the staging.

Fatal Complications

Approximately 60,000 patients die annually due to pressure ulcer complications. Wound-related bacteremia increases mortality to 55%.

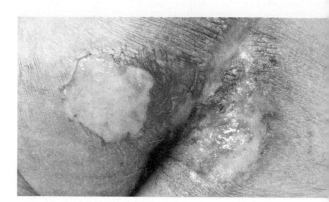

FIGURE 12-5 Extensive pressure ulcer on the buttocks and coccyx with bleeding.
© RJ22/Shutterstock

Stage	Clinical Presentation	Signs and Symptoms
TABLE 12-1 Pressure Ulcer Staging		
Stage I	• Nonblanching erythema (red patch)—no blanching, or whitening, when site is briefly compressed with a finger • Skin is intact—damage is to capillaries beneath the epidermis	• Pain
Stage II	• Blister or shallow open wound at site • Damage to the epidermis and dermis	• Pain • Bleeding
Stage III	• Shallow wound extends to the subcutaneous layer • Damage to all three layers of skin • Fat is visible at the base of the wound	• Pain • Bleeding • Cellulitis • Sepsis
Stage IV	• Muscle or bone can be seen at the base of the wound • Damage extends through skin to underlying tissues	• Osteomyelitis

Stages of Pressure Sores

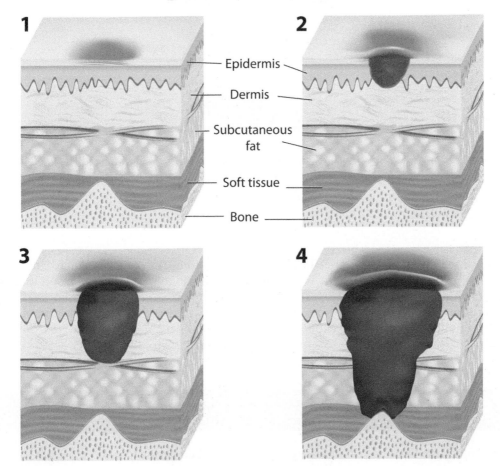

FIGURE 12-6 Extent of damage to the layers of skin during the four stages of pressure ulcers.

© Alila Medical Media/Shutterstock

Assessment and Treatment

When performing your secondary survey, thoroughly inspect the patient for pressure ulcers (**FIGURE 12-7**). Keep in mind that a patient may have been moved prior to your arrival, so pressure ulcers may not be found on the dependent side of the patient. Assess any pressure ulcers found by noting the stage, location, appearance, and size of the ulcer, along with the condition of surrounding body structures.

Prevention is the primary focus in patients at risk of pressure ulcers. Decrease pressure on bony sites by providing extra padding, such as the traction splint thigh support system, ischial pad, or the ischial perineum cushion, to any firm surface the patient must remain in contact with. If a rigid spine board must be used, lay a blanket between the board and the patient to prevent shearing forces that can occur while extricating the patient. EMS practitioners are well positioned to assist patients with pressure ulcer prevention through educating patients, family, and caregivers on how ulcers develop and possible complications.

Treatment involves removing pressure from the site and managing the open wound as any other. Manage

Pressure Ulcer Wound Care

- Stage 1: Gently wash with soap and water or rinse with normal saline. Pat dry area and dress with dry, sterile bandages. Remove pressure.
- Stage 2: Rinse with normal saline (lightly flushing open sores). Pat dry and cover with dry, sterile dressings. Remove pressure.
- Stages 3 and 4: Rinse and flush the area, removing any loose necrotic tissue. Gently dry the area and cover with sterile dry dressings. Remove pressure.

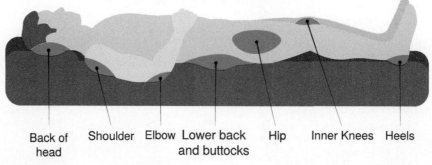

Pressure sores often form over bony
prominences in fixed patients

Back of head | Shoulder | Elbow | Lower back and buttocks | Hip | Inner Knees | Heels

FIGURE 12-7 Common sites of pressure ulcers.

© Raccoonez/Shutterstock

bleeding with localized direct pressure. Bleeding may persist longer than expected if the patient is taking anticoagulant medication. Treatment can also include pain relief. Consider reducing doses of opiates (if used) in older adult patients due to decline in liver function.

During transport, prolonged immobilization without additional padding can result in tissue necrosis and ulceration as well as increased pain and discomfort in the older patient. Therefore, complications from skin breakdown must be considered during the transport and immobilization of older patients.

CASE STUDY

You and your partner are working for an emergency ambulance service in an urban area. You are dispatched to a mobile home for a welfare check on a 72-year-old male who is not answering his phone. It is a hot summer day. The air temperature is 98°F (36.6°C).

QUESTIONS

- What is your differential diagnosis?
  - The complaint is unknown, so almost anything is possible. Assume the worst-case scenario and prepare for a resuscitation. Given the environmental conditions, heat-related illness is also very possible. The rest of your differential diagnosis include:
    - Stroke
    - Hypoglycemia
    - Dehydration
    - Infection
    - Anemia
    - Toxins
    - Seizure
    - Tumors
    - Malnutrition
    - Elder maltreatment
- How does the patient's age affect your assessment approach?

  - You decide to incorporate the GEMS diamond into your assessment.

When you arrive at the scene, you see that law enforcement is present. An officer comes out of the home to meet you. She explains that she and her partner gained entry through an unlocked front door and found the patient in his bed. She says the patient is awake and needs medical attention. She tells you, that according to the neighbors, the patient is being cared for by his intellectually disabled son. The patient was also receiving home care, but the neighbors haven't seen the nurse's car for 5 days. The neighbors became concerned after not seeing any movement at the house recently, so they called emergency services.

With law enforcement already on scene, you deem the scene safe and don your routine personal protective equipment (PPE). You enter the home and immediately note the strong smell of urine and feces. The home is very warm with only fans being used for cooling. No air-conditioning appears to be present. The home is untidy and dirty dishes are piled in the kitchen sink. The law enforcement officer leads you to the patient, who is lying in a hospital bed in the living room. There are no sheets on the vinyl mattress, and the patient is wearing pajamas.

Another law enforcement officer and the patient's son are standing beside the bed. The patient cannot accomplish activities of daily living (ADLs) by himself due to a stroke he suffered 6 months prior. His son provides meals and medications and tells you that his dad has "a lady" who takes care of him, but she hasn't been there "in a while."

Your initial impression of the man is that he is alert and interacting with the law enforcement officer, though his responses to questions are somewhat confused and disoriented. He has no apparent difficulty breathing, and his color is good. He tells you he feels "weak all over."

You perform a primary survey and find the following:

- X–No hemorrhage noted.
- A–Airway is patent.
- B–Breathing is normal. Lungs are auscultated and are clear bilaterally.
- C–Radial pulses are strong; skin is warm and dry and normal color.
- D–GCS is 14 (E4, V4, M6), pupils are 5, equal, and reactive.
- E–Open wound noted at coccyx, skin tears at upper arms; no rash or edema found.

QUESTIONS

- What is the cardinal presentation and the chief complaint?
  - Cardinal presentation is the patient's medical problem: Welfare check
  - Chief complaint is what the patient complains of: N/A in this case

- Are any interventions required before assessment can continue?
  - Given the ambient temperature and the increased risk of heat-related illness is older patients, you

should provide a cooler environment for the patient before continuing.

- Does this patient require immediate transport, or can you remain on scene and continue your assessment?
  - You decide to remain on scene and continue your assessment.

- Are there other assessments you would like to perform besides the standard assessments?
  - Not at this time.

You are concerned that the patient has altered mental status, is bedridden, and too warm. The altered mental status can indicate heat exhaustion. Given the warmth in the room and the speed at which older adult patients can deteriorate, you decide to move the patient from the home to the air-conditioned ambulance before continuing with your assessment.

Once in the cooler environment of the ambulance, your partner assesses vital signs while you consult the patient for the OPQRST and SAMPLER information.

- O–Gradual
- P–Feels much better in the cooler environment
- Q–Generalized weakness
- R–None
- S–5/10
- T–1 week

- S–General weakness
- A–NKDA
- M–May not be compliant for the last 5 days with citalopram, atorvastatin, clopidogrel, gabapentin, propranolol, lisinopril
- P–Hypertension, depression, hyperlipidemia, stroke with residual left-sided weakness, atrial fibrillation
- L–Ate soup 2 hours ago
- E–Home care nurse not visiting, temperature in home too warm
- R–Age, immobility, history of stroke

Vital Signs

- HR: 110, irregular
- SpO$_2$: 95% room air
- RR: 16
- BP: 130/90
- Temp: 98.6°F (37°C) tympanic
- ETCO$_2$: 40 mm Hg
- BGL: 88 mg/dl (4.9 mmol/l)

A 12-lead ECG is unremarkable except for atrial fibrillation.

A physical head-to-toe assessment is performed, and you note the patient has dry mucous membranes, left-sided weakness due to a previous stroke, skin tears on both lower arms, and a stage II pressure ulcer at the coccyx with redness and warmth.

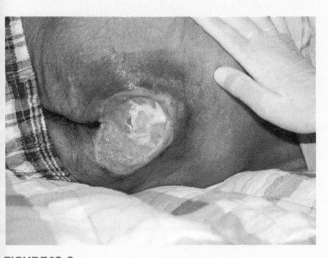

FIGURE 12-8

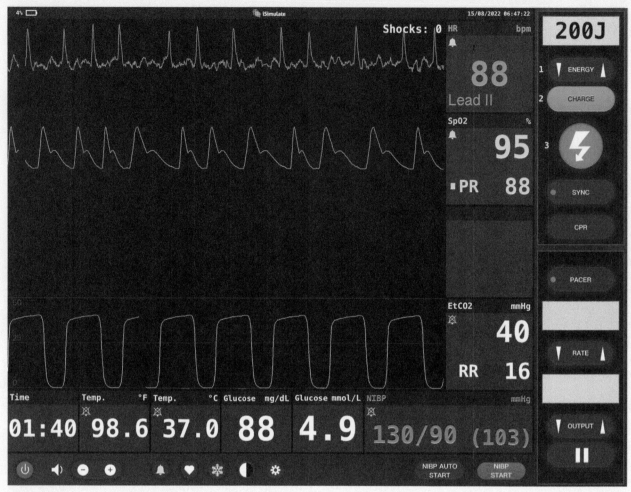

FIGURE 12-9

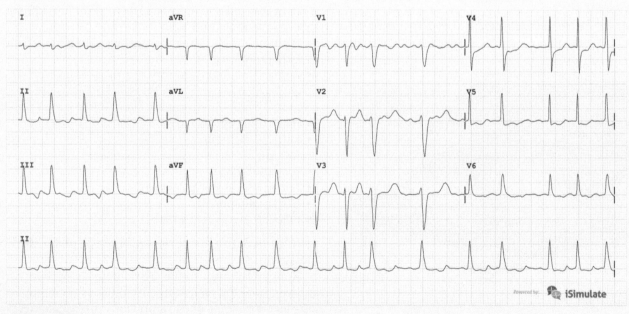

FIGURE 12-10

Detailed Physical Exam

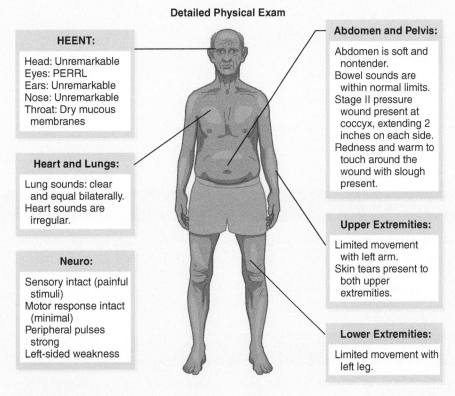

HEENT:

Head: Unremarkable
Eyes: PERRL
Ears: Unremarkable
Nose: Unremarkable
Throat: Dry mucous
  membranes

Heart and Lungs:

Lung sounds: clear
  and equal bilaterally.
Heart sounds are
  irregular.

Neuro:

Sensory intact (painful
  stimuli)
Motor response intact
  (minimal)
Peripheral pulses
  strong
Left-sided weakness

Abdomen and Pelvis:

Abdomen is soft and
  nontender.
Bowel sounds are
  within normal limits.
Stage II pressure
  wound present at
  coccyx, extending 2
  inches on each side.
Redness and warm to
  touch around the
  wound with slough
  present.

Upper Extremities:

Limited movement
  with left arm.
Skin tears present to
  both upper
  extremities.

Lower Extremities:

Limited movement with
  left leg.

FIGURE 12-11

GEMS DIAMOND REVIEW

Geriatric Assessment: The patient has age-related changes expected for a 72-year-old, as well as disability from a stroke.

Environmental Assessment: His residence is not sanitary, is warm with no air-conditioning, and food quality and amount are both questionable.

Medical Assessment: Patient may not have been compliant with medications for the past 5 days; daily home care has not visited for the last 5 days; patient is not receiving appropriate care for his condition based on wounds found.

Social Assessment: The patient is unable to perform ADLs and is totally reliant on his adult son, who is intellectually disabled.

QUESTIONS

- How will you treat the patient?
  - Place in position of comfort.
  - Give IV therapy/fluid bolus.
  - Bandage patient wounds with dry sterile dressing as time permits.

- What are your goals for this patient?
  - Transport to the most appropriate ED for wound care management.
  - Communicate with home health agency to identify why they have not come and address patient findings.
  - Monitor patient for any changes.

- What conditions are part of your potential differential diagnosis now?
  - Decubitus ulcer to coccyx
  - Dehydration
  - Infection
  - Anemia
  - Toxins
  - Malnutrition

- Where is the most appropriate treatment destination and why?
  - This patient should be transported to the closest appropriate facility.

Treatment

- BLS
  - Place in position of comfort.
  - Monitor vitals.
  - Bandage skin tears and pressure wound.

- ALS
  - BLS care
  - IV therapy/fluid bolus

- Critical care
  - BLS/ALS care

You begin transport to the local hospital after his wounds are dressed. He is transported in side-lying position to avoid further pressure on his coccyx. You administer a fluid bolus. You continuously monitor the patient's ECG and mental status. There are no changes en route.

CASE STUDY WRAP-UP

Once at the hospital, the patient is assessed for dehydration and his medication prescriptions are resumed. He is then admitted and receives wound care. A home care case worker is assigned and determines that his home health care was accidentally cancelled when the agency involved changed management. The patient was later discharged to a long-term care facility.

CHAPTER WRAP-UP

Skin is the body's number one defense against infection. The aging population is already at high risk for infection due to a compromised immune system. Weakened skin adds to their risk.

When assessing older adult patients who have medical complaints and mobility issues, conduct thorough head-to-toe examinations to identify all wounds as you would a trauma patient.

Prevention of pressure ulcers is the primary goal when managing patients at increased risk of this type of injury.

REFERENCES

Epidemiology of melanoma and nonmelanoma skin cancer—the role of sunlight. In: Reichrath J, eds. *Sunlight, Vitamin D and Skin Cancer. Advances in Experimental Medicine and Biology.* Vol 624. Springer, NY; 2008.

Gallegos Hernández JF, Nieweg OE. [Cutaneous Melanoma (CM): Current Diagnosis and Treatment]. *Gac Med Mex.* 2014;150 Suppl 2:175–182.

Leonardi GC, Falzone L, Salemi R, et al. Cutaneous melanoma: from pathogenesis to therapy (Review). *Int J Oncol.* 2018;52(4):1071–1080. doi: 10.3892/ijo.2018.4287

Linos E, Chren M-M, Covinsky K. Geriatric dermatology: a framework for caring for older patients with skin disease. *JAMA Dermatol.* 2018;154(7):757–758. doi:10.1001/jamadermatol.2018.0286

Lomas A, Leonardi-Bee J, Bath-Hextall F. A systematic review of worldwide incidence of nonmelanoma skin cancer. *Br J Dermatol.* May 2012;166(5):1069–1080.

Marieb E, Hoehn K. *Human Anatomy and Physiology.* 9th ed. Pearson Education; 2013.

National Institute on Aging. Skin Care and Aging. Last reviewed October 1, 2017. Accessed September 28, 2022. https://www.nia.nih.gov/health/skin-care-and-aging

Sanders M, McKenna K. *Sanders' Paramedic Textbook.* 5th ed. Jones and Bartlett Learning; 2019.

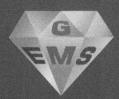

CHAPTER 13

Ventilators

LESSON OBJECTIVES

- Differentiate between invasive and noninvasive ventilation.
- Identify the types of mechanical ventilators.
- Review the basic ventilatory modes and parameters of a ventilator.
- Recall the DOPE mnemonic for patients who receive ventilator support.

Introduction

Ventilations must be provided for patients unable to maintain adequate spontaneous breathing. Manual ventilators (e.g., bag-valve mask [BVM] devices) were originally developed to provide this support, followed by the creation of mechanical ventilators. Once limited to use in intensive care units, ventilatory technology has improved and now much smaller and lighter models can be used outside the hospital setting (**FIGURE 13-1**). This development has led to an increase in the use of mechanical ventilatory support by EMS and provided an opportunity for ventilated patients to live in the general community. In addition, positive-pressure mechanical ventilation has been shown to save more lives when compared to positive-pressure manual ventilation. As in the hospital, EMS patient care goals include improving airway patency, ventilation, and oxygenation.

Familiarity Is Not Competency

Remember that familiarity with ventilators is not the same as competency in their use.

Invasive Mechanical Ventilation

Mechanical ventilation can be provided invasively or noninvasively. **Invasive ventilation** is provided through

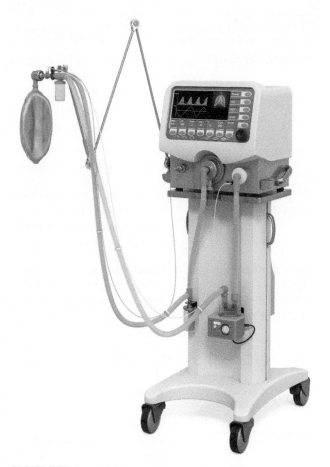

FIGURE 13-1 Artificial, or mechanical, ventilator.
© AlexLMX/Shutterstock

an endotracheal or tracheostomy tube. Advantages of this type of ventilation are that higher ventilation pressures can be used without fear of gastric inflation and it can be used on any patient, specifically patients unable to cooperate with manual ventilation (e.g., patients with altered mental status). Because advanced airways are used, the advantages of airway patency and deep suctioning can be included on this list.

Disadvantages of invasive ventilation include the risk of ventilator-acquired pneumonia, ventilation-induced lung injury, and difficulty weaning the patient off mechanical ventilation. The use of an invasive airway increases the risk of trauma to the upper airway, esophageal intubation, potential need for induction medications, and increased risk for tracheal stenosis.

Noninvasive Mechanical Ventilation

Noninvasive mechanical ventilation does not use an advanced airway. Ventilations are provided through a mask over the mouth and nose or nose alone.

Advantages of this style of ventilation are that it can be instituted without delay or premedication, and it can be easily stopped or paused. Because an advanced airway is not used, it preserves the airway defenses against infection and allows the patient to communicate verbally.

Disadvantages of this style of ventilation are that it can only be used if the patient is cooperative and can tolerate the mask pressure and noise; airflow can dry oral, nasal, and optic membranes; it can cause insomnia; and pressure ulcers from the mask can occur.

Mechanical Ventilator Types

TABLE 13-1 lists different types of mechanical ventilation.

Ventilator Settings

TABLE 13-2 shows common ventilator settings (**FIGURE 13-4**).

TABLE 13-1 Mechanical Ventilators	
Type of Ventilator	**Description**
Volume ventilator	■ Provides a preset volume of gas with each cycle ■ Delivers a consistent tidal volume ■ Does not change with airway resistance or compliance of the thorax and lungs ■ Stops the flow (with a safety release valve) if the volume reaches too high of an airway pressure
Pressure ventilator	■ A pressure-controlled device stops inspiration once a preset pressure level is met ■ Commonly used in patients with airway resistance that is unlikely to change
Negative-pressure ventilator	■ Lifts the rib cage and lowers the diaphragm, creating negative air pressure in the lungs to draw in air ■ Could be used in patients lacking muscular ability to inhale ■ Includes settings for the ventilation rate and the pressure of negative force being used
Continuous positive airway pressure (CPAP) (FIGURE 13-2)	■ Used in patients who are breathing spontaneously and whose airways collapse on exhalation, such as those with obstructive sleep apnea ■ Maintains higher air pressure within the airways to prevent airway collapse—in other words, it keeps the airways inflated ■ Maintains the same pressure during inspiratory and expiratory phases ■ Keeping airways open during exhalation increases the alveolar surface area available for respiration and therefore increases oxygenation
Bilevel positive airway pressure (BiPAP) (FIGURE 13-3)	■ An alternative to CPAP for patients who need additional support with spontaneous breathing ■ Provides two levels of air pressure: a relatively higher air pressure during inhalation, called the inspiratory positive airway pressure, and relatively lower air pressure during exhalation, referred to as the expiratory positive airway pressure ■ Stents airways open as with CPAP, but also assists inspiration

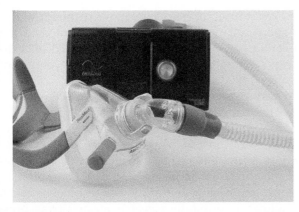

FIGURE 13-2 Continuous positive airway pressure (CPAP) machine with face mask.
© Susan Edmondson/Shutterstock

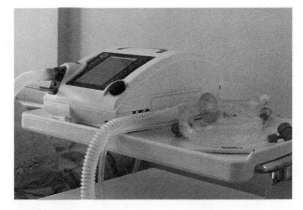

FIGURE 13-3 Bilevel positive airway pressure (BiPAP) machine with face mask.
© Zhitnikov Vadim/Shutterstock

TABLE 13-2 Ventilator Settings	
Setting	**Description**
Respiratory rate	■ Number of ventilations delivered over 1 minute ■ Usually set between 10 and 14
Tidal volume	■ Volume of air delivered with each ventilation ■ Set at approximately 6 to 8 ml/kg of ideal patient weight ■ Setting may be reduced in patients with poor lung compliance to avoid lung injury due to high pressures developing during inflation
Fraction of inspired oxygen	■ Expressed as a decimal ■ Percentage of oxygen in the gas inhaled ■ Written as FiO_2 ■ Settings range from 0.21 to 1 ■ Titrate to lowest amount needed to maintain target arterial saturation
Peak flow	■ Speed at which the tidal volume is delivered ■ Settings range from 35 to > 100 L/min
Inspiratory expiratory ratio	■ Refers to the duration of the inspiration to the duration of expiration ■ Written as I:E ■ Normal breathing involves twice the duration of exhalation than inhalation and would be written as 1:2 ■ Patients with asthma would require longer expiratory times to avoid air trapping and lung injury, so their I:E may be 1:3 or 1:4
Inspiratory time	■ Length of time over which inspiratory flow, or tidal volume, will be delivered
High-pressure alarm	■ Warning to ventilator operator that pressure being used to deliver tidal volume is exceeding the set limit ■ Usually set to 10 cm H_2O higher than peak inspiratory pressure
Low-pressure alarm	■ Warning to ventilator operator that pressure within the ventilator circuit is lower than set tolerance and the ventilator may not be able to generate the pressure needed to ventilate the patient ■ Typically indicates a large leak or disconnect in the ventilator circuit ■ Usually set to 5 to 10 cm H_2O lower than the peak inspiratory pressure
Peak inspiratory pressure	■ The peak pressure generated during ventilation ■ This value should never exceed 40 cm H_2O or the lungs may be injured by over-inflation

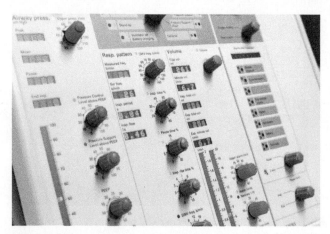

FIGURE 13-4 Ventilator settings panel.
© toysf400/Shutterstock

Mechanical Ventilation Modes

There are various types of mechanical ventilation modes so that the ventilations delivered can be optimized for the type of patient receiving care. The assist control (A/C) mode is usually used to ventilate long-term ventilator patients. This mode will ventilate the patient a set number of times per minute to a set tidal volume. If the patient breathes spontaneously between the ventilations, then the ventilator will assist the spontaneous breath by providing the set tidal volume. This setting is ideal for respiratory muscle recovery since the ventilator does all the work. There is a risk of hyperventilation if the patient attempts spontaneous breathing too often.

The synchronized intermittent mandatory ventilation (SIMV) mode provides a set number of breaths to a set volume while allowing the patient to breath spontaneously. A spontaneous breath is not assisted by the ventilator. This mode allows the patient to gradually

---

take over control of their ventilations without the risk of hyperventilating. This mode is well suited to the recovering patient who needs to be weaned off ventilatory support. SIMV can be done with volume or pressure.

Airway pressure release ventilation (APRV) mode allows the patient to breath spontaneously. When the patient is not breathing, an inverse I:E ratio is applied. In other words, instead of a short period of high inspiratory pressure followed by a longer period of exhalation, this mode uses a long period of high inspiratory pressure followed by a shorter period of exhalation. This allows a constantly elevated mean airway pressure, which allows better oxygenation. This mode works well for patients with acute lung injury, acute respiratory distress, atelectasis, and severe COVID-19.

DOPE Mnemonic

Patients receiving positive-pressure ventilation by mechanical ventilators must be constantly monitored. Any change in a patient's status requires immediate assessment and troubleshooting of any problems. The **DOPE mnemonic** was developed to guide the ventilator operator efficiently through such a troubleshooting process (**TABLE 13-3**).

Primary Modes

The two primary modes for ventilators are A/C and SIMV.

Breathe First!

If the mechanical ventilator is not functioning properly, disconnect the ventilator circuit from the endotracheal tube and provide manual ventilations with a bag-valve mask device before troubleshooting the ventilator.

Critical Thinking Question

Why is it important to note the tracheal tube number at the lips prior to transferring an intubated patient onto your stretcher for transport?

TABLE 13-3 DOPE Mnemonic

Mnemonic	Meaning
D	Dislodgement of the endotracheal tube ▪ Assess the depth of the tube. ▪ Identify where the tube is at the lip line and where it is supposed to be. ▪ Evaluate ETCO$_2$ and lung sounds. ▪ Assess for symmetrical chest expansion. ▪ Evaluate gastric sounds. ▪ Replace tube if it has become dislodged.
O	Obstruction ▪ Evaluate bag-valve mask device compliance. ▪ Assess for lung sounds. ▪ Inspect the endotracheal tube for mucus or blood. ▪ Assess the endotracheal tube for pinching or bending. ▪ Clear the obstruction by suctioning or straightening tubing, sedate patient if biting the tube.
P	Pneumothorax ▪ Evaluate bag-valve mask device compliance. ▪ Assess and compare equality of lung sounds. ▪ Assess pulse oximetry, hypotension, jugular vein distension. ▪ Tracheal deviation is a late finding and may not be detectable. ▪ Decompress the affected side with needle thoracostomy.
E	Equipment ▪ Evaluate power source—plugged in, battery power remaining. ▪ Inspect tubing for kink or pinching. ▪ Inspect oxygen supply for disconnection or cylinder depletion. ▪ Assess oximetry and capnometry for function. ▪ Switch to bag-valve mask device while troubleshooting equipment, take corrective action on equipment as needed.

CASE STUDY

You are dispatched to a long-term care facility to transport a 67-year-old female with decreased SpO$_2$. She requires evacuation due to a heavy storm approaching with a significant risk of flooding the facility. The patient has a tracheostomy and is ventilator dependent. It is a warm, spring morning. The air temperature is 71°F (21.7°C).

QUESTIONS

- What are your initial concerns?
  - Given the environmental conditions, speed of evacuation is of concern given that the patient must use a ventilator.

- What is your differential diagnosis?
  - Because this case involves evacuation of a patient, potential differential diagnoses are not required.

- How does the patient's age affect your assessment approach?
  - Due to the patient's age, you decide that you will include the GEMS approach to your assessment.

When you arrive on scene, you are met by a staff member who directs you to the patient, who is lying in bed, sharing a room with two additional patients. You determine the scene is safe and that you are wearing the appropriate personal protective equipment (PPE).

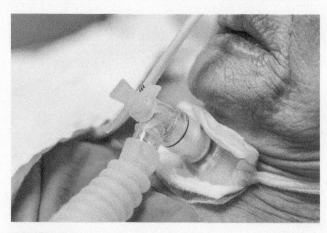

FIGURE 13-5

© PongMoji/Shutterstock

As you make your way to the patient, you note the room is cluttered with patient belongings. You note the patient has a tracheostomy tube and is ventilator dependent. No odors are noted, and she appears to have appropriate food and needed supplies. The temperature in the room is cool.

The staff advises you that the patient has been ventilator dependent and residing at their facility for a year. The staff further advises that an alarm was going off on the patient's ventilator indicating decreased SpO_2. Staff then obtained an SpO_2 with an alternate finger probe and it confirmed the patient has a decreased SpO_2 at 89%.

She is being transported to a facility 45 miles (72 km) away that can care for a ventilator-dependent patient. The patient's daughter visits daily and will meet her mother at the receiving facility. The staff provide you with medical records and patient medications in a packet.

You perform a primary survey and find the following:

- X–No obvious hemorrhage.
- A–Obstructed, with minimal air movement noted through the tracheostomy.
- B–Rapid and regular with increased work of breathing. Lung sounds are diminished bilaterally.
- C–Radial pulses are rapid, strong, and regular, capillary refill time brisk. Skin is warm and dry.

Pretransport Check

A proper assessment of your patient is just as important when taking over patient care to transfer a patient from one facility to another as it is when you are responding to a medical or trauma call. Before assuming care of a patient, ensure you are familiar with the patient's medical history, including the care they are receiving currently. In this lesson, we will focus on the pretransport checks required for an intubated patient on a mechanical ventilator.

Ensure the patient is breathing adequately by assessing oximetry, capnometry, capnography, and blood pressure. Match your transport ventilator settings to the settings of the nontransport bedside model. Settings will vary from patient to patient, but common settings include the following:

- Mode: A/C and SIMV/Volume are the most common modes.
- Rate: 12 ventilations per minute is considered normal but often ranges from 10 to 14.
- Tidal volume: Based on a ratio of ml per kg of ideal body weight of the patient, often 500 ml for an adult.
- Positive end expiratory pressure (PEEP): 5 cm H_2O is the normal starting point and then titrated to effect.
- I:E ratio: 1:2 is the normal ratio.
- Fraction of inspired oxygen (FiO_2): 35% is the typical starting point and then titrated to effect.

- Sensitivity: –1 cm H_2O is the typical setting and is the pressure the patient must generate to trigger a breath.
- High-pressure alarm: 40 cm H_2O.
- Low-pressure alarm: 10 cm H_2O.
- Power source: Internal battery, additional external battery, and inverter cord
- Equipment: Irrigation saline packets, French suction catheters, working suction device, enough oxygen for the duration of the stretcher portion of the transport, bag-valve mask device

Before transferring the patient over to your stretcher, ensure the endotracheal tube is properly secured and there is enough slack in the ventilator tubing to allow for the move. The safest transfer utilizes at least three care practitioners: one controlling the head and ventilator tubing, and one on each side of the patient's torso. Larger patients will require more care practitioners. All movement should be coordinated by the practitioner at the patient's head.

Once the patient has been placed and secured on the stretcher, re-confirm the endotracheal tube placement, and ensure that the ventilator circuit has not been trapped or pinched under the patient or trailing on the floor. Make sure the transport ventilator and oxygen cylinder are properly secured to the stretcher before moving.

- D–Alert.
- E–Lying in bed; no rashes, edema, or lacerations noted.

QUESTIONS

- What is the cardinal presentation and the chief complaint?
  - Cardinal presentation is the patient's medical problem: Respiratory distress, tracheostomy tube obstruction.
  - Chief complaint is what the patient complains of: Decreased SpO_2.
- Are there any life threats identified in this case?
  - Yes: Respiratory distress and possible airway obstruction.
- Are any interventions required before assessment can continue?
  - You need to determine the cause of the possible airway obstruction, which requires your regular assessments to be performed.

- What are the transport considerations?
  - Whether to transfer the patient to the agency's transport ventilator and transport, or to transport the patient on their ventilator; ensuring adequate supplies for the duration of the transport.

Once in the ambulance, you assess vital signs while you consult the patient for the OPQRST and SAMPLER assessments.

- O–Unknown
- P–None
- Q–None
- R–None
- S–None
- T–13 minutes
- S–Decreased SpO_2, tracheostomy tube obstruction, diminished lung sounds, increased work of breathing, facility transfer
- A–NKDA
- M–COPD, MI × 3, NIDDM, hypertension, and heart failure

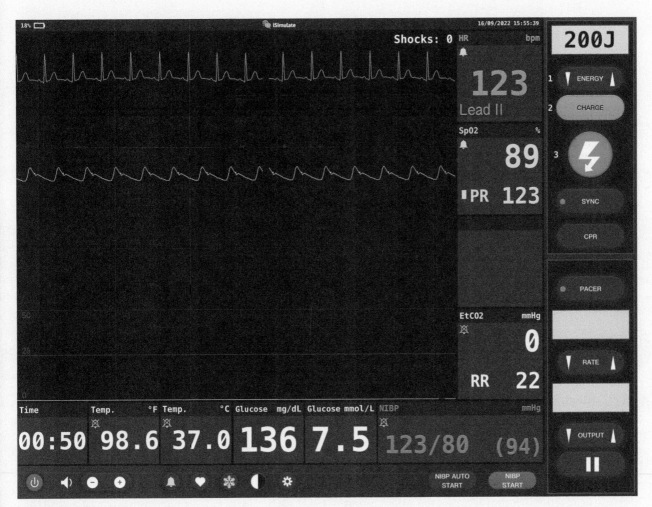

FIGURE 13-6

Detailed Physical Exam

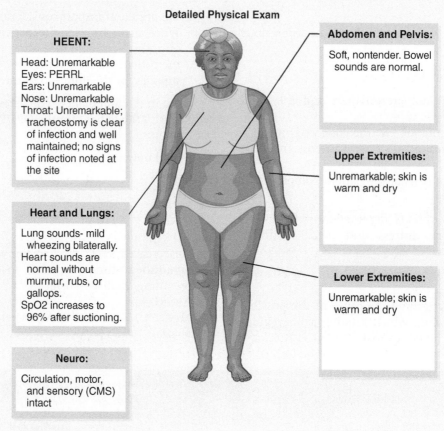

HEENT:

Head: Unremarkable
Eyes: PERRL
Ears: Unremarkable
Nose: Unremarkable
Throat: Unremarkable; tracheostomy is clear of infection and well maintained; no signs of infection noted at the site

Heart and Lungs:

Lung sounds- mild wheezing bilaterally. Heart sounds are normal without murmur, rubs, or gallops.
SpO2 increases to 96% after suctioning.

Neuro:

Circulation, motor, and sensory (CMS) intact

Abdomen and Pelvis:

Soft, nontender. Bowel sounds are normal.

Upper Extremities:

Unremarkable; skin is warm and dry

Lower Extremities:

Unremarkable; skin is warm and dry

FIGURE 13-7

Copyright © 2024 National Association of Emergency Medical Technicians (NAEMT).

- P–Prednisone, albuterol, ipratropium bromide, hydrochlorothiazide, metformin, furosemide, potassium, nitroglycerin
- L–Continuous water for the last 2 hours
- E–Ventilator alarm noting a decrease in SpO_2; being relocated due to an evacuation
- R–Tracheostomy and ventilator dependent, age

Vital Signs

- HR: Elevated
- SpO_2: 89% on ventilator
- $ETCO_2$: Unable to obtain initially; after suctioning, it is 36 mm Hg with normal waveform

- RR: Increased and improves to 18 after suctioning
- BP: Normal
- Temperature is normal
- BGL: 136 mg/dl (7.5 mmol/l)
- Cardiac monitor reveals sinus tachycardia
- 12 lead was not assessed during transport

A physical head-to-toe assessment is performed and you note the tracheostomy is clear of infection and well maintained with no infection noted at the site, but plugged with mucus. The patient has mild wheezing bilaterally and heart sounds are normal. You clear the mucus plug with suction. Her SpO_2 increases to 96% after suctioning.

 GEMS DIAMOND REVIEW

 Geriatric Assessment: The patient is a 67-year-old female with consistent age-related changes.

 Environmental Assessment: Room is cluttered with patient belongings, without significant obstacles. No odor noted, appears to have appropriate food and needed supplies. Temperature in the room is cool.

Medical Assessment: The patient has a tracheostomy and is ventilator dependent. The staff advise you the patient is compliant with her meds and received her medication for this morning.

 Social Assessment: The patient requires assistance to accomplish ADLs. She lives in a long-term care facility with two room-mates. Her daughter visits daily.

QUESTION

- What are your goals for this patient?
  - Improve and maintain oxygenation; goal is 94–99% as measured by pulse oximetry.
  - The patient's tracheostomy obstruction should be cleared, and the patient transported in a position of comfort.

During the first few minutes of transport, the patient's oxygen saturation drops to 75% and the patient becomes slightly diaphoretic and anxious. You use the DOPE mnemonic to identify potential ventilator problems and how they would be managed with this patient. As you work through the DOPE mnemonic, you find the main oxygen tank is empty. The oxygen tank was low and not checked by the crew at the beginning of the shift. The tank provided oxygen initially, but it quickly ran out. Luckily, the crew had four spare full M-15 (D cylinder) portable oxygen tanks on the ambulance to use for transport.

CASE STUDY WRAP-UP

After switching to the portable oxygen tanks, the patient's SpO2 rose back to 96% and remained stable for the duration of transport to the receiving facility. At the receiving facility, the patient was met by her daughter and staff. The severe storm caused flooding to the patient's previous facility, leading to long-term closure for repairs. The patient was transported back to the previous facility after 3 months.

CHAPTER WRAP-UP

The most common mechanical ventilator modes that EMS will encounter are A/C and SIMV/V. EMS practitioners must be familiar with the basic concepts of ventilators and their functions. However, having a basic understanding of ventilators only makes you better prepared to assist a fully trained ventilator operator. The DOPE mnemonic is a very useful tool to quickly troubleshoot ventilation issues.

REFERENCES

Guérin C, Lévy P. Easier access to mechanical ventilation worldwide: an urgent need for low-income countries, especially in face of the growing COVID-19 crisis. *Eur Respir J.* 2020;55(6). doi:10.1183/13993003.01271-2020

Mazoff S, Bird K. Synchronized Intermittent Mandatory Ventilation. StatPearls [Internet]. Updated January 2022. Accessed June 22, 2022. https://pubmed.ncbi.nlm.nih.gov/31751036/

Mora Carpio AL, Mora JI. Ventilator Management. [Updated 2022 Mar 27.] In: StatPearls [Internet]. Treasure Island (FL): StatPearls Publishing; 2022 Jan. https://www.ncbi.nlm.nih.gov/books/NBK448186/

Pinto V, Shrma S. Continuous Positive Airway Pressure. StatPearls [Internet]. Updated May 2, 2022. Accessed on June 22, 2022. https://www.ncbi.nlm.nih.gov/books/NBK482178/

Rahmanzade R, Rahmanzadeh R, Tabarsi P, et al. Noninvasive versus invasive ventilation in COVID-19 once size does not fit all! *Anesth Analg.* 2020;131(2):e114-e115.

Scottish Intensive Care Society. No date provided. Accessed on June 22, 2022. https://www.scottishintensivecare.org.uk/training-education/sics-induction-modules/ventilation-i-e-ratio/

Sembroski E, Sanghavi D, Bhardwaj A. Inverse ratio ventilation. StatPearls [Internet]. Updated April 12, 2022. Accessed June 22, 2022. https://www.ncbi.nlm.nih.gov/books/NBK535395/

Swindin J, Sampson C, Howatson A. Airway pressure release ventilation. *BJA Educ.* 2020 Mar;20(3):80–88.

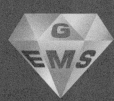

CHAPTER 14

Urinary Catheter and Colostomy Bag Care

LESSON OBJECTIVES

- Discuss the purposes and indications for a urinary catheter and colostomy bag.
- Identify urinary catheter and colostomy bag complications.
- Discuss the management of a patient with a urinary catheter and a colostomy bag.

Introduction

Providing health care in the community is a good alternative to hospital-based care in certain cases and conditions. Studies show patient prognosis improves when a patient can be properly managed outside the hospital setting. Subsequently, qualified patients, some of whom have implanted medical devices, are discharged from the hospital with home healthcare visits as part of their discharge plans.

Consequently, EMS contact with patients wearing implanted medical devices is increasing. Familiarization with these devices, as well as how to assess, manage, and transport patients wearing them, is important for EMS practitioners. Two common implanted devices, the urinary catheter (**FIGURE 14-1**) and the colostomy bag (**FIGURE 14-2**), are discussed in this lesson.

Urinary Catheter

Older adult patients may have urinary dysfunction due to age-related changes in the urinary system (such as urinary retention due to prostate enlargement in men, and incontinence and nocturnal voiding in men and women due to urinary sphincter dysfunction). To manage this dysfunction, indwelling urinary catheters are provided for some patients (**FIGURE 14-3**). Indwelling urinary catheters can be placed through the urethra or the abdominal wall. Urethral urinary catheters,

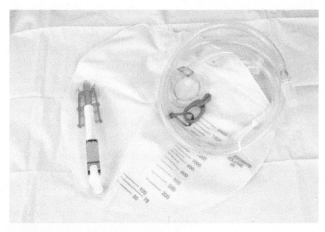

FIGURE 14-1 Urinary catheter.
© MedstockPhotos/Shutterstock

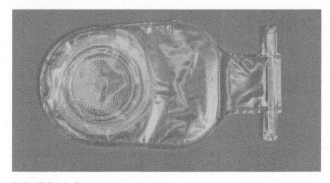

FIGURE 14-2 Colostomy bag.
© Butus/Shutterstock

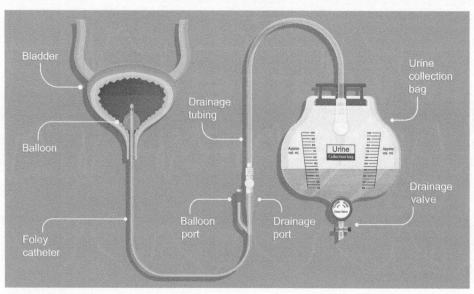

FIGURE 14-3 Components of a urinary catheter.

TABLE 14-1 Foley Catheter Urinary Collection System

Element	Description
Foley catheter	■ Soft flexible tubing inserted through the urethra into the bladder to allow drainage ■ Proximal end has a fluid-filled balloon that seals closed the bladder outlet and holds catheter in place ■ Distal end has two ports: one to instill sterile saline into the catheter balloon and the other to drain urine
Drainage tubing	■ Flexible clear tubing that connects the drainage port of the catheter to the collection bag ■ Long enough to allow patient movement while keeping collection bag below the level of the bladder ■ Has a clamp to facilitate catheter change
Collection bag	■ Collapsible bag that attaches to the drainage tubing ■ Calibrated to estimate volume of urine within the bag ■ Clear to allow macroanalysis of the urine ■ Includes a drainage port to drain bag as required ■ Has the ability to connect to frame of hospital bed or stretcher

also referred to as Foley catheters, are the most common type (**TABLE 14-1**). These devices include a flexible hollow tube inserted through the urethra to the urinary bladder. They come in various sizes and are selected to best suit the size of the patient to prevent urethral injury. Suprapubic urinary catheters are surgically inserted through the abdominal wall and into the urinary bladder.

Indications

The primary indications for the placement of a Foley catheter in older adults include management of the following:

- Acute urinary retention or bladder outlet obstruction
- Incontinence in palliative or hospice care patients
- Perioperative or critically ill patients

Foley catheters may be placed in males to relieve urinary retention due to obstructed urethral flow caused by prostate enlargement. Less commonly, females may develop a urethral obstruction due to complications from surgery to correct incontinence. Foley catheters are also placed to monitor the kidney function of a critically ill or injured patient. In the absence of renal illness or failure, urine production is a good indicator of end-organ perfusion and so is an effective measure of a patient's circulatory status.

Other indications for the insertion of a Foley catheter include immobility of the patient, obtaining a urine sample from a patient who cannot voluntarily void, assisting healing in patients with incontinence and open sacral or peritoneal wounds, instilling medical dye for an imaging study, and to improve patient comfort as part of end-of-life care. This type of catheter should be replaced at least every 3 months.

A suprapubic catheter is used as an alternative to the Foley catheter when the latter is not feasible (e.g., if the urethra is damaged or blocked). This type of catheter should be replaced every 4 to 6 weeks.

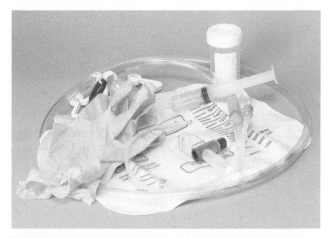

FIGURE 14-4 Sterile supplies required for placement of a urinary catheter.
© MedstockPhotos/Shutterstock

Critical Thinking Question

Why must sterile saline be instilled into the catheter balloon and not air like on an advanced airway cuff?

Catheter Insertion

Although the process of placing a urinary catheter is not complicated, patients may feel anxious at the prospect of catheter placement. Aseptic technique is essential to minimize the risk for catheter-associated urinary tract infection (CAUTI; **FIGURE 14-4**). Despite specialized training required to ensure aseptic technique, CAUTI is the most common complication of Foley catheter use. Specific training on catheter insertion in older adult patients is required due to the patient's normal age-related changes.

Older adult male patients are more difficult to catheterize due to normal urethral positioning complicated by an enlarged prostate. Identification of the urinary meatus is more challenging due to anatomic changes common to older adult female patients.

Catheter Complications

Catheterized patients who are ambulatory may find their activities of daily life (ADLs) are restricted. Others may find their enjoyment and participation in social activities are reduced. However, a properly sized, inserted, and secured catheter should not interfere greatly with the patient's day-to-day activities.

In addition to infection, other medical complications of catheterization include:

- Catheter blockage due to mineral deposits on the catheter
- Allergic reaction
- Bladder stones
- Urethral injury, pain, and bladder spasms

UTIs and Catheterization

Urinary tract infection (UTI) is the most common complication of urinary catheterization. A study showed that out of 125 catheterized patients, 22.4% developed symptomatic UTI and 52.8% developed bacterial colonies on the tip of the catheter.

Mechanical complications with catheterization include:

- Drainage tube occlusion due to kinking or entrapment in a folding stretcher carriage
- Backflow of urine up the drainage tubing due to elevation of the collection bag above the level of the patient's bladder
- Blockage of urine flow by a full collection bag
- Catheter balloon deflation causing catheter dislodgement
- Bladder lining being sucked into the catheter tip by negative pressure due to the collection bag sitting too low below the patient's bladder

The catheter may also be inadvertently removed with the inflated balloon. This can occur due to any of the following:

- Patients with dementia or delirium pulling out the catheter
- Excessive straining during bowel movements
- Bladder spasms
- Catheter being pulled by the collection bag being dropped or entangled in bedding, clothing, or other equipment

Inadvertent removal with an inflated balloon can cause significant injury to the entire length of the urethra.

Complications can also occur following a medical catheter removal by a caregiver. The complications that can develop within days of removal include:

- UTI
- Urine leakage
- Bladder spasms
- Difficulty starting and stopping urine flow
- Sexual dysfunction

Catheters can dislodge due to balloon deflation or trauma (pulled). In case of dislodgement:

- Follow local protocols regarding either removing the dislodged catheter or securing it in place during transport.
- Never attempt to put the same catheter back in.
- Sterile technique is required, so a new catheter is the only option.
- Patient should be transported to the ED so potential internal damage can be assessed/treated.

Catheter Care

The initial assessment of a patient with a urinary catheter should include an assessment of the urinary collection system. Ensure the collection bag is not leaking, is not full, and there is no blood in the urine. If the collection bag needs to be emptied prior to transport from a medical facility, advise the nursing staff as they will likely need to document the volume of urine emptied (**FIGURE 14-5**).

Specific considerations for catheter care depend on the complication involved:

- UTI—Treat according to local protocol, transport.
- Sepsis—Treat according to local protocol, transport.
- Allergic reactions—Treat as required, depending on severity of allergic reaction and as per local protocol; transport.
- Pain—Ensure the catheter is not under pressure/being pulled, offer analgesia (if appropriate under local protocol), transport.

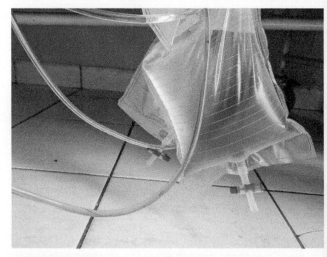

FIGURE 14-5 Full urine collection bag.
© Haelen Haagen/Shutterstock

- Catheter bag issue—Raise if too low, lower if too high, empty if too full; monitor for resolution of symptoms; transport if required.
- Blood in urine—Multiple potential causes, including infection and trauma; cause needs to be established. Provide supportive care, oxygen (if necessitated by SpO_2), fluids (if necessary/indicated under local protocol), and transport.
- Encrustations/blockage—If local protocols allow for clearing, do so. If not, but local protocols allow for replacing catheter, do so. If not, transport patient.

Transport Considerations

- After moving the patient to your stretcher, ensure the drainage tubing is not pinched or bent and the collection bag is secured to the stretcher below the level of the patient's bladder.
- Never leave the collection bag on top of the patient, as this increases the risk of infection.
- During transport, monitor the patient for any complications from the urinary collection system such as pain and pressure build-up in the bladder, indicating lack of urine flow.
- If the patient complains of pain, ensure that nothing is pulling on the drainage tube and correct as necessary.
- If the patient complains of bladder discomfort, assess the drainage tubing for obstruction, such as kinked or pinched tubing or closed tube clamp.

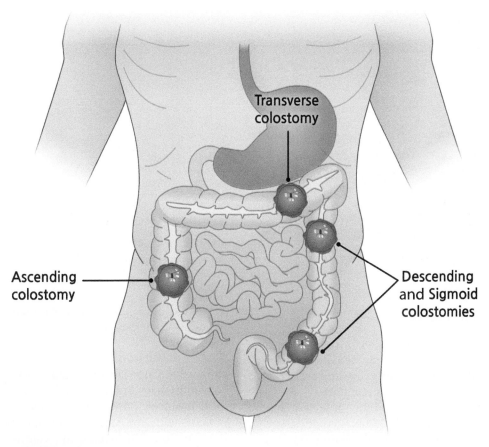

Transverse
colostomy

Ascending
colostomy

Descending
and Sigmoid
colostomies

FIGURE 14-6 Colostomy locations.
© ddoll/Shutterstock

Colostomy Bag

A colostomy is a surgical opening in the abdominal wall that communicates with the colon to allow fecal excretion (**FIGURE 14-6**). A colostomy may be permanent or temporary depending on the reason it was needed. Indications for a permanent colostomy include ulcerative colitis, Crohn disease, diverticulitis, irritable bowel syndrome, colorectal cancer, nonfunctioning anal sphincter, or bowel obstructions.

A colostomy bag, or pouching system, is a medical device designed to adhere to the abdominal skin, creating an airtight and watertight seal around the **stoma**, to collect feces (**FIGURE 14-7**). Pouching systems can include a flange that attaches to the skin and a pouch that attaches to the flange or a one-piece system in which the bag attaches directly to the skin. A reusable colostomy bag (drainable pouch) has a drainage port with a clamping system, while others are intended for single use (closed-end pouch) and therefore have no drainage capacity. However, even a reusable bag should be replaced with a new one every 3 to 4 days due to the possibility of a build-up of bacteria.

Replacing a Colostomy Bag

Do not attempt to empty or replace colostomy bags unless trained to do so and allowed by local protocol.

1. Use hand hygiene procedures.
2. Ease the pouch away from the stoma, being careful not to pull on the stoma (consider using adhesive remover if required).
3. Either dispose of the entire pouch and contents into the appropriate disposal bag or empty the contents into a toilet first and then dispose of the pouch into the appropriate disposal bag.
4. Use warm water and soap (preferably mild) to clean the stoma and surrounding area, then dry.
5. On the new bag, remove the protective cover from the flange.
6. Secure the flange over the stoma while ensuring that there are no creases or twists in the bag/flange.
7. Dispose of any waste appropriately.
8. Use hand hygiene procedures again.

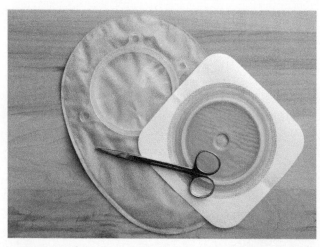

FIGURE 14-7 Colostomy supplies.
© Margaret M Stewart/Shutterstock

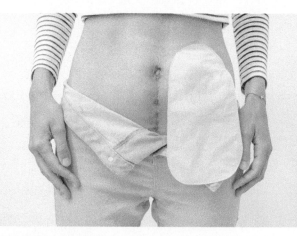

FIGURE 14-8 Colostomy bag on a patient's abdomen.
© Branimir Todorovic/Shutterstock

Complications

Colostomy bags are designed to be inconspicuously worn under clothing (**FIGURE 14-8**). Smaller bags are available for daytime use to be even more discreet. Despite the potential for social discomfort or embarrassment, colostomy bags should not interfere with most ADLs and most activities. Certain activities, such as extreme contact sports, risk dislodging the bag. **TABLE 14-2** describes complications that are associated with colostomies.

Management

When managing a patient with a colostomy bag, note if the patient has any pain at the site. Inspect the stoma for any swelling, bleeding, tissue protrusion, blockage, signs of skin irritation or discoloration, and signs of poor hygiene. Ensure there is no tension or pulling on the colostomy bag, it is not twisted, and it is not more than half full. If the patient is nonemergent, have the patient or their caregiver empty or replace the bag prior to transport.

Note any abnormalities and manage the patient with supportive care. Do not attempt to empty or replace colostomy bags unless trained to do so and allowed by local protocol. Provide pain relief as necessary. Some patients with new stoma sites will call EMS after cleaning the stoma by wiping too vigorously, causing minor abrasions and bleeding. While not life-threatening, these patients should be transported for wound cleaning and further education on stoma care.

No Pressure

When transporting a patient with a colostomy bag, *be careful not to put pressure on the bag when moving the patient or positioning them on the stretcher.*

TABLE 14-2 Complications Associated with Colostomies		
Complication	**Description**	**Treatment**
Pain	■ Depends on cause	■ Treat with supportive care, offer analgesia (if appropriate under local protocol), transport
Parastomal hernia	■ Protrusion of abdominal contents through the incision in the abdominal wall made to create the stoma ■ Most common surgical complication associated with colostomies	■ Treat with supportive care, transport

Complication	Description	Treatment
Prolapse of bowel wall	■ Bowel wall protrudes through the stoma opening	■ Treat with supportive care, transport
Colostomy bag blockage	■ Obstruction of the colostomy pouch opening by tissue or fecal matter	■ Treat with supportive care, transport
Skin irritation	■ Caused by skin reaction to the adhesive, drying of skin by adhesive, poor hygiene, or friction caused by pouch rubbing against the skin	■ Treat with supportive care, transport
Retraction	■ Stoma withdrawing back into the abdominal cavity	■ Treat with supportive care, transport
Ischemia	■ Lack of blood flow to part of the intestinal wall	■ Treat with supportive care, transport
Dislodged colostomy bag	■ Caused by adhesive failure or traumatic removal	■ Treat with supportive care, transport
Blood in fecal matter	■ Multiple potential causes, including infection and trauma ■ Cause needs to be established	■ Provide supportive care, oxygen (if necessitated by SpO$_2$, fluids (if necessary/ indicated under local protocol), transport

Copyright © 2024 National Association of Emergency Medical Technicians (NAEMT).

CASE STUDY

It is 1400 on a warm, spring afternoon. The air temperature is 71°F (21.7°C). You and your partner are staffing an emergency response ambulance and are dispatched to the home of a 77-year-old male who is complaining of pelvic pain.

The scene appears safe as you don your personal protective equipment (PPE) while approaching the house. You are met at the door by the patient's wife. She leads you to her husband who is lying in bed in his bedroom. The house is tidy, warm, and free of obstacles

QUESTIONS

- What is your differential diagnosis?
  - Cancer
  - Muscle strain
  - Sexually transmitted infection
  - Urinary tract infection
  - Appendicitis
  - Hernia
  - Kidney stones
  - Gastrointestinal problems (e.g., IBS)
  - Urinary catheter complications
- How does the patient's age affect your assessment approach?
  - You decide to include the GEMS Diamond as part of your overall assessment because of his age.

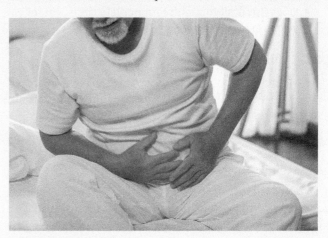

FIGURE 14-9

© 220 Selfmade studio/Shutterstock

and odors. When you enter the bedroom, you notice he has a walker. You decide that the scene is safe and you have on the appropriate PPE.

The patient is a heavy-set, older adult man who is alert and interactive, breathing normally, and has pale skin. As you approach the patient, the wife advises you that they have lived together in the same house for 40 years. They live independently except for a public health nurse who visits once a month.

The wife decided to call EMS because her husband has been complaining of pelvic pain since the morning, and his catheter collection bag has been empty. She says this is unusual, as it would normally need to be emptied by now. The patient tells you his catheter has been in place for 12 weeks.

You perform a primary survey with the following results:

- X–No obvious hemorrhage noted.
- A–Patent airway.
- B–Breathing is regular and unlabored with adequate depth. Lung sounds are clear bilaterally.
- C–Radial pulses are strong and regular; skin is cool and dry to touch.
- D–Oriented to self, place, and time; pupils are equal and reactive.
- E–No signs of trauma, edema, or rash.

QUESTIONS

- What is the cardinal presentation and the chief complaint?
  - Cardinal presentation is the patient's medical problem: Pelvic pain, oliguria
  - Chief complaint is what the patient complains of: Pelvic pain

- Are any interventions required before assessment can continue?
  - No interventions are required at this time.

- Does this patient require immediate transport, or can you remain on scene and continue your assessment?
  - You decide it is safe to remain on the scene and continue your assessment.

- What further assessments would you like to perform?
  - No additional assessments beyond the standard assessments are needed at this time.

You direct your partner to collect vital signs while you assess the patient's history using the OPQRST and SAMPLER mnemonics:

- O–Sudden
- P–Worsens when attempting to sit up or stand up

- Q–Feels like pressure
- R–None
- S–6/10 and constant
- T–6 hours

- S–Pelvic pain, oliguria
- A–NKDA
- M–Patient states he is compliant with finasteride prescription
- P–Benign prostate enlargement, Foley catheter in place
- L–Dinner last night, no appetite today
- E–Onset this morning, nothing unusual yesterday, denies trauma
- R–Age, prostate enlargement, indwelling catheter

Vital Signs

- HR: 74
- RR: 16
- BP: 114/76
- SpO$_2$: 98% on room air
- ETCO$_2$: 42 mm Hg
- Temp: 97.6°F (36.4°C)
- BGL: 100 mg/dl (5.6 mmol/l)

A 12 lead is unremarkable, showing a normal sinus rhythm.

Your secondary body survey identifies that he has suprapubic tenderness and firmness on palpation.

- **HEENT**:
  - Head: Unremarkable
  - Eyes: PERRL
  - Ears: Unremarkable
  - Nose: Unremarkable
  - Throat: Unremarkable

- **Heart and Lungs:**
  - Lung sounds: clear bilaterally. Heart sounds are normal without murmur, rubs, or gallops.

- **Neuro:**
  - Circulation, motor, and sensory (CMS) intact

- **Abdomen and Pelvis:**
  - Firm, tender on palpation. Bowel sounds are normal. Pelvic pain.

- **Upper Extremities:**
  - Unremarkable

- **Lower Extremities:**
  - Unremarkable

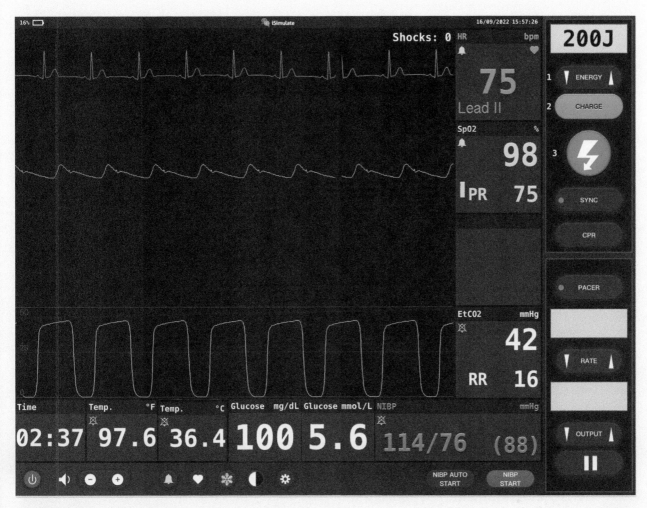

FIGURE 14-10

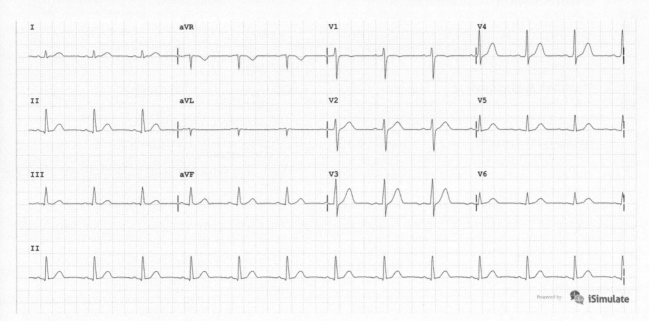

FIGURE 14-11

Detailed Physical Exam

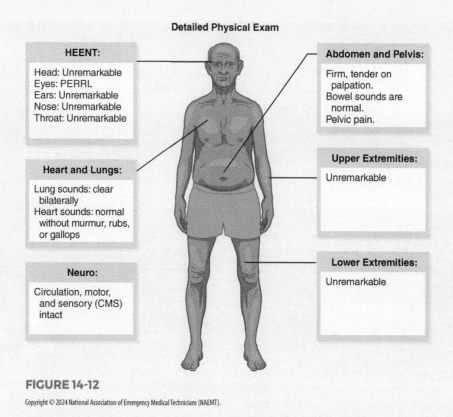

HEENT:

Head: Unremarkable
Eyes: PERRL
Ears: Unremarkable
Nose: Unremarkable
Throat: Unremarkable

Abdomen and Pelvis:

Firm, tender on
    palpation.
Bowel sounds are
    normal.
Pelvic pain.

Heart and Lungs:

Lung sounds: clear
    bilaterally
Heart sounds: normal
    without murmur, rubs,
    or gallops

Upper Extremities:

Unremarkable

Neuro:

Circulation, motor,
    and sensory (CMS)
    intact

Lower Extremities:

Unremarkable

FIGURE 14-12

Copyright © 2024 National Association of Emergency Medical Technicians (NAEMT).

GEMS DIAMOND REVIEW

 Geriatric Assessment: 77-year-old with expected age-related changes

 Environmental Assessment: Home is well-kept, warm, no odors, and seems safe and comfortable with no obstacles. Patient appears well fed and not to be lacking anything.

 Medical Assessment: Compliant with medications, catheter is replaced every 3 months, goes to medical appointments.

 Social Assessment: Independent and lives full time with his wife, has 1 monthly home care visit.

Treatment

- BLS
  - Place in position of comfort.
  - Monitor vitals.

- ALS
  - BLS care
  - Consider pain management
  - Catheter replacement

- Critical care
  - BLS/ALS care

QUESTIONS

- What does differential diagnosis include now?
  - Muscle strain
  - Urinary tract infection
  - Hernia
  - Kidney stones
  - Gastrointestinal problems (irritable bowel syndrome [IBS])
  - Urinary catheter complications

- What prehospital treatment should be provided?
  - Treat patient with supportive care.
  - Apply oxygen and treat pain, if needed.
  - Consider replacing the catheter (if trained and allowed by protocol).

– Monitor the patient for any changes during transport.
- What is the most appropriate treatment destination?
  – The patient should be transported to the closest appropriate facility.

The patient is transported in the Fowler position on a stretcher to the closest appropriate facility. The patient declines your offer of analgesia. The patient is monitored during transport and there are no changes on arrival at the ED.

CASE STUDY WRAP-UP

At the hospital, the catheter is replaced, and 1.2 L of urine is drained. The catheter is assessed, and it is noted that it has been obstructed with mineral encrustation. Given the amount drained, the patient is monitored for hypotension and positioned supine. He is assessed for a UTI and bladder injury, and it is determined he has neither. At the hospital, he and his wife are counseled on proper hygiene and management of a urinary catheter. The couple is advised to replace the urinary catheter every 8 weeks to avoid encrustation. The patient is discharged home into his wife's care, and a follow-up appointment is made with the patient's primary care provider.

CHAPTER WRAP-UP

With the increasing older adult population and the prevalence of urethral obstruction due to prostate disorders, EMS practitioners can anticipate encountering patients in the community with indwelling catheters.

Gastrointestinal (GI) disorders are also common in this age group so increased exposure to patients with colostomy bags should also be expected.

Understanding these medical devices and the complications associated with them will help the EMS practitioner offer optimal care to their patients. Effectively managing a patient with a urinary catheter or colostomy bag will help prevent further complications.

REFERENCES

American Cancer Society. Types of colostomies and pouching systems. ACS website. Last updated October 2019. Accessed June 25, 2022. https://www.cancer.org/treatment/treatments-and-side-effects/treatment-types/surgery/ostomies/colostomy/types-of-colostomies.html

Bhatia N, Daga MK, Garg S, et al. Urinary catheterization in medical wards. *J Glob Infect Dis*. 2010 May;2(2):83–90.

Centers for Disease Control and Prevention. Catheter-associated urinary tract infections. Last reviewed October 16, 2015. Accessed April 5, 2021. https://www.cdc.gov/hai/ca_uti/uti.html

Centers for Disease Control and Prevention. Catheter-associated urinary tract infections (CAUTI). Last reviewed November 5, 2015. Accessed April 5, 2021. https://www.cdc.gov/infectioncontrol/guidelines/cauti/index.html

Lee EA, Malatt C. Making the hospital safer for older adult patients: a focus on the indwelling urinary catheter. *Perm J*. 2011 Winter; 15(1):49–52. doi: 10.7812/TPP/10-067

Murken D, Bleier J. Ostomy-related complications. *Clin Colon Rectal Surg*. 2019;32(03):176–182. doi:10.1055/s-0038-1676995

National Health Service. Types of urinary catheter. NHS website. Last updated February 2020. Accessed on June 23, 2022. https://www.nhs.uk/conditions/urinary-catheters/types/#:~:text=A%20suprapubic%20catheter%20is%20used,bag%20strapped%20to%20your%20leg

Rodrigues FP, Novaes JAV, Pinheiro MM, Martins P, Cunha-Melo JR. Intestinal ostomy complications and care. *Gastrointestinal Stomas*. Published online October 23, 2019. doi:10.5772/intechopen.85633

Saint S, Trautner BW, Fowler KE, et al. A multicenter study of patient-reported infectious and noninfectious complications associated with indwelling urethral catheters. *JAMA Intern Med*. 2018;178(8):1078–1085. doi:10.1001/jamainternmed.2018.2417

Stylinski R, Alzubedi A, Rudzki S. Parastomal hernia—current knowledge and treatment. *Wideochir Inne Tech Maloinwazyjne*. 2018 Mar;13(1):1–8.

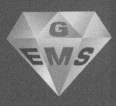

CHAPTER 15

Implantable Cardioverter Defibrillators

LESSON OBJECTIVES

- Analyze ECG findings in patients with ventricular dysrhythmias, paced rhythms, and implantable cardioverter defibrillators (ICDs).
- Describe the special concerns of an older patient with an ICD.

- Identify the signs and symptoms of a patient with a malfunctioning ICD.
- Discuss the management of patients with ICDs.

Introduction

The purpose of an implantable cardioverter defibrillator (ICD) is to treat potentially fatal ventricular cardiac rhythms. An ICD uses defibrillation to treat ventricular fibrillation (V-fib) and asynchronous cardioversion to treat ventricular tachycardia (V-tach). An ICD can also provide demand pacing therapy for dangerous bradycardias and overdrive pacing therapy to treat potentially lethal supraventricular tachycardias. More recent ICDs can also provide **cardiac resynchronization therapy (CRT)** to treat heart failure. All therapies are accomplished through the placement of electrodes in the atrial and ventricular myocardium (**FIGURE 15-1**).

What's in a Name?

The first generations of implantable cardiac therapy devices were limited to the demand pacemaker mode, and so took on the name "pacemaker." These devices are now much more sophisticated and provide multiple therapies, but are still often referred to as pacemakers by some older patients.

Indications and Risks

The indications for surgical placement of an ICD include (**FIGURE 15-2**):

- Secondary prevention in patients with a history of sustained V-fib or V-tach
- Resuscitation from sudden cardiac death thought to be due to V-fib or V-tach
- Prevention of cardiac arrests in patients at risk of developing V-fib or V-tach
- Patients with symptomatic bradycardia or prolonged sinus arrest arrythmias
- Patients with recurrent supraventricular tachycardias refractory to other therapies
- Patients with heart failure

Long-term risks of an ICD include:

- Infection
- Erosion of the device
- Lead failure due to mechanical stress placed on the lead (**FIGURE 15-3**)
- Inappropriate heart rhythm detection with subsequent countershock
- Battery depletion
- Electronic failure of the device

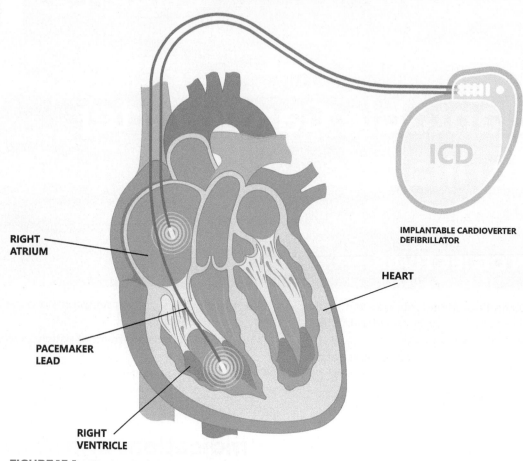

RIGHT
ATRIUM

PACEMAKER
LEAD

RIGHT
VENTRICLE

IMPLANTABLE CARDIOVERTER
DEFIBRILLATOR

HEART

FIGURE 15-1 ICD placement and components.
© Pepermpron/Shutterstock

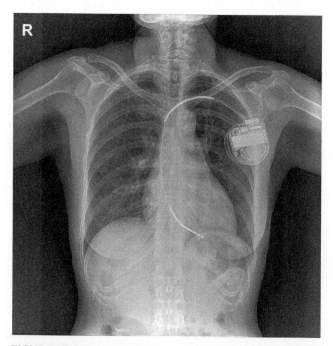

FIGURE 15-2 Radiograph showing ICD placement and leads.
© April stock/Shutterstock

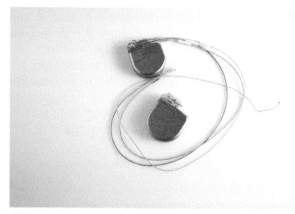

FIGURE 15-3 ICDs with leads.
© Logtnest/Shutterstock

Depression, Anxiety, and Phantom Shocks

Studies have shown that patients have a decrease in the quality of life in the first year after surgery and are prone to anxiety and depression if the ICD has

ctivated. The more often the ICD cardioverts the pa-
ent, the worse the anxiety and depression become.
atients you treat may be suffering severe anxiety, as
eir ICD has activated, and need therapeutic commu-
ication and assurance from you.

Some patients report the sensation of **phantom
hocks**. The cause of this phenomenon is unknown,
ut these patients require the same management as
ose in whom the ICD has activated, as phantom
hocks can only be differentiated from a cardioversion
ent after the ICD data has been downloaded and
CG rhythm interpreted.

A Shocking Experience

Up to 87% of ICD patients suffer anxiety and 33%
suffer depression. Originally thought to be caused
by receiving an ICD countershock, anxiety and
depression are more likely due to the knowledge
that a life-threatening condition exists and events
are occurring.

Reliable functioning of the ICD depends on proper
ensing of the electrical activity of the heart. Earlier
CD models used a unipolar lead and may not have
een shielded enough from electromagnetic interfer-
nce. Since 2010, ICDs utilize more reliable bipolar
ad placement and are better shielded. Risk is low for
lectromagnetic interference caused by cell phones and
ther smaller, personal devices (e.g., iPod or similar de-
ice). However, there may still be potential interference
om larger equipment such as metal detectors, high
oltage lines, and industrial equipment. The American
eart Association offers guidance on their website for
atients with ICDs (www.heart.org/en/health-topics
arrhythmia/prevention--treatment-of-arrhythmia
evices-that-may-interfere-with-icds-and-pacemakers).

Recognition

atients with ICDs will often wear medical ID brace-
ts or tags indicating they have an implanted medical
evice. The ICD is placed beneath the skin, so its out-
ne is apparent on inspection of the left upper chest
FIGURE 15-4). When operating in the pacing function,
e ECG will present with thin negative spikes preced-
ng a QRS complex with a widened and altered mor-
hology similar to a preventricular contraction. The
untershock in defibrillation or synchronized cardio-
ersion mode will present with a lethal rhythm fol-
wed by a tight, large amplitude displacement from
e isoelectric line. This will be followed by a brief
systolic pause and then return of a stable rhythm.

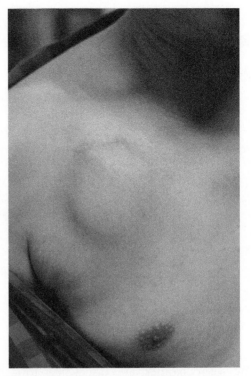

FIGURE 15-4 Patient with ICD. Note the outline of the ICD
on the right upper chest directly under the clavicle.
© Chaikom/Shutterstock

Inappropriate countershocks will present with the displacement occurring on top of a stable rhythm.

Management

If you witness the patient going into cardiac arrest, allow the ICD to sense and discharge. If there is no response to the ICD, then follow normal resuscitation
procedures. The ICD is typically placed under the skin
on the anterior chest inferior to the left clavicle. To
avoid damage to the ICD and ensure the countershock
you are delivering is not blocked by the ICD, ensure
your defibrillator pads or electrodes are at least 4 inches
(10 cm) from the ICD. Anterior-posterior placement
may be used instead of anterior-lateral defibrillation
pad placement.

If the ICD is administering inappropriate shocks, a
medical magnet can be placed above the ICD to pause
its function. The ICD will remain paused as long as the
magnet is in place. Be prepared to manage arrythmias
while the ICD is paused.

Following an event, the ICD events and ECG
rhythms can be downloaded by the patient's cardiologist. More current models can transmit event and ECG
histories remotely. Whenever an ICD has provided a
countershock, the patient must be transported to an
appropriate medical facility.

CASE STUDY

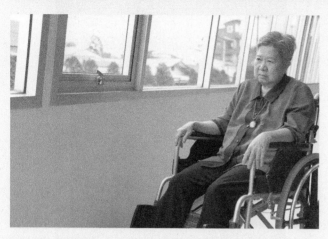

FIGURE 15-5 Your patient is sitting in her wheelchair in her room. She is anxious and worried.

© 88studio/Shutterstock

You and your partner are dispatched to a local assisted-living facility for ICD activation. An 85-year-old female is complaining of palpitations, and two sudden, sharp, stabbing pains in her chest. She was in the dining room of the facility when this episode occurred. She was returned to her room and 911 was activated.

QUESTIONS

- What is your differential diagnosis?
  - Tachycardic arrhythmia
  - Anxiety
  - Acute myocardial infarction (AMI)
  - Medication overdose (e.g., digoxin)
  - ICD malfunction

- How does the patient's age affect your assessment approach?
  - You decide that you will include the GEMS approach to your assessment due to the patient's age.

You arrive at the front entrance of the facility and are met by facility staff who lead you to the patient's room. The facility is clean, well lit, and has no odors, and the hallways are free of obstacles. When you get to the patient's room you find her awake and sitting in a wheelchair; her breathing seems normal, and her skin is cool, dry, and has normal color (**FIGURE 15-5**). You notice that she wears glasses and uses a cane. Her room is tidy and very warm. You assess that the scene is safe, and you are wearing the correct PPE.

The facility nurse is standing beside the patient. She tells you that while the patient was in the dining room waiting for lunch, she began feeling palpitations. She then screamed twice after feeling two episodes of

sudden, sharp, stabbing pain in her chest. She was very anxious after this episode, so she was returned to her room where the nurse has been trying to calm her.

The nurse hands you a copy of the patient's health information. You skim through the notes and find a valid advance care directive that instructs EMS that only comfort care is desired. The patient wishes that care be limited to pain relief, passive oxygenation, and bleeding control. The nurse also tells you that the patient can perform activities of daily living (ADLs) independently and has a sister who visits twice a week.

You perform a primary survey and find the following:

- X–No hemorrhage noted.
- A–Airway is patent.
- B–Breathing is normal. Lungs are auscultated and are clear bilaterally.
- C–Radial pulses are strong, irregular, and fast; capillary refill time is < 3 seconds; skin is cool and dry and normal color.
- D–GCS is 15 (E4, V5, M6); pupils are 5, equal, and sluggish.
- E–No wounds, rash, or edema found.

QUESTIONS

- What is the cardinal presentation and the chief complaint?
  - Cardinal presentation is ICD discharges.
  - Chief complaint is palpitations just prior to ICD discharges, then chest pain post ICD discharges.

- Are there any life threats with this patient?
  - There are several potential life threats:
    o Ventricular arrhythmia
    o Patient could be defibrillated into life-threatening arrhythmia or cardiac arrest.
    o Possible reoccurrence of multiple inappropriate discharges of ICD.

- Does this patient require immediate transport or can you remain on scene and continue your assessment?
  - You decide it is safe to remain on scene and proceed with a detailed assessment. You immediately attach an ECG monitor.

- What does differential diagnosis include now?
  - Ventricular arrhythmia
  - AMI
  - Angina
  - Muscular skeletal pain
  - Inappropriate ICD shock delivery

You immediately attach the ECG monitor to determine if the ICD is functioning normally. You assess the patient's cardiac rhythm to be atrial fibrillation and confirm with her medical information that this is normal for her.

Your partner assesses vital signs while you consult the patient and her medical notes for the OPQRST and SAMPLER assessments.

- O–Sudden
- P–Resolved after two presumed countershocks from ICD
- Q–"Fluttering" sensation at substernal chest
- R–None
- S–1/10
- T–10 minutes

- S–Episode of palpitations
- A–Aspirin
- M–Staff state she is compliant with metoprolol, atorvastatin, losartan, and warfarin
- P–AMI, atrial fibrillation, hyperlipidemia, noninfarction cardiomyopathy, ICD placed 10 years ago
- L–Ate breakfast this morning

- E–Facility staff said she had no prodromal symptoms prior to sitting down for lunch
- R–Age, severe heart disease

You note that her medical chart includes history of nonischemic cardiomyopathy and left ventricular ejection fraction (LVEF) of 38%. LVEF is the measurement of how much blood is being pumped out of the left ventricle of the heart with each contraction. A normal LVEF is 55–70%; however, for this patient, an LVEF of 38% means that 38% of the total amount of blood in the left ventricle is pumped out with each beat. Typically, an LVEF of less than 40% indicates heart failure.

Her vital signs (**FIGURE 15-6**) are as follows:

- HR: 110, irregular
- SpO$_2$: 97% room air
- RR: 16
- BP: 126/84
- Temp: 97.6°F (36.4°C)
- ETCO$_2$: 40 mm Hg
- BGL: 82 mg/dl (4.6 mmol/l)

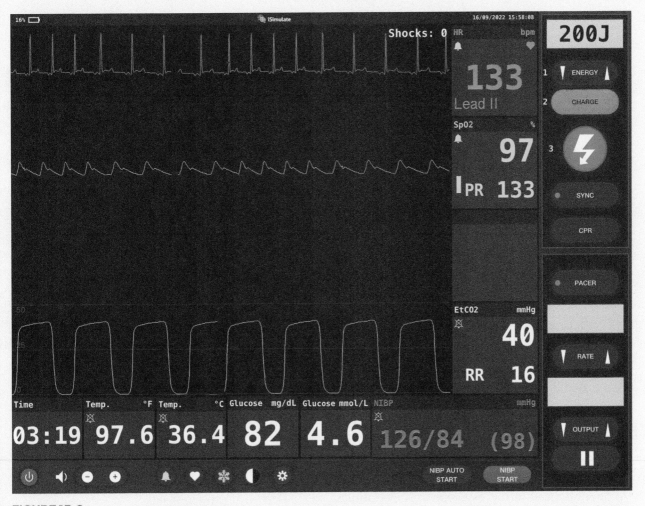

FIGURE 15-6

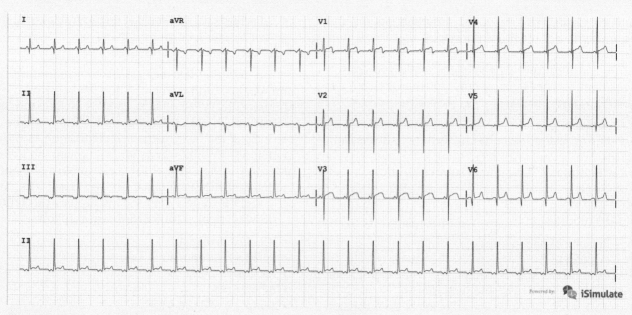

FIGURE 15-7

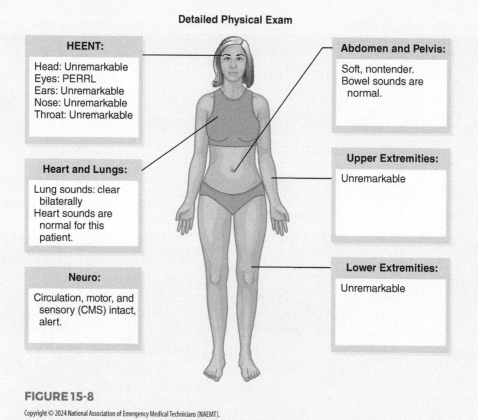

FIGURE 15-8

The 12-lead ECG shows a variable rapid response rate of 90–110 with no acute ST segment changes.

- 12 lead ECG shows pathologic Q waves in V2, V3, V4; hypertrophic R waves (**FIGURE 15-7**)

A physical head-to-toe assessment is performed, and no new findings were noted.

- **HEENT**
  - Head: Unremarkable
  - Eyes: PERRL
  - Ears: Unremarkable
  - Nose: Unremarkable
  - Throat: Unremarkable

- **Heart and Lungs**
  - Lung sounds: clear bilaterally. Heart sounds are normal for this patient.
- **Neuro**
  - Circulation, motor, and sensory (CMS) intact, alert.

- **Abdomen and Pelvis**
  - Soft, nontender. Bowel sounds are normal.
- **Upper Extremities**
  - Unremarkable
- **Lower Extremities**
  - Unremarkable

GEMS DIAMOND REVIEW

 Geriatric Assessment: The patient has age-related changes expected for an 85-year-old plus patient with advanced heart disease

 Environmental Assessment: Her residence appears safe and well maintained; she uses a cane for assistance with ambulation and wears glasses; no odors; appears neat and clean; temperature in apartment is very warm

 Medical Assessment: Patient states she is compliant with medications and appointments and there have been no recent prescription changes. History of nonischemic cardiomyopathy and left ventricular ejection fraction (LVEF) of 38%.

 Social Assessment: The patient is independent and relies on staff for medication administration, visited by sister twice a week.

Treatment

- BLS
  - Place in position of comfort.
  - Check glucose.
  - Monitor vitals.

- ALS
  - BLS care
  - IV therapy
  - 12-lead ECG
  - Continuous cardiac monitoring
- Critical care
  - BLS/ALS care

QUESTIONS

- What would your initial treatment be?
  - Care for patients whose ICDs have activated is largely supportive; these patients must be seen by a cardiologist whenever the ICD provides a countershock. Monitor the ECG and remain alert for any changes/patient deterioration, and provide assurance and emotional support during transport.
  - Treatment should also be focused on:
    - Interpretation of possible ventricular arrhythmia
    - Determination of inappropriate discharge of ICD
    - Use of a donut magnet to temporarily shut off the shock-therapy functions of the device if heart rate accelerates and patient complains of palpitations once again

- What treatment should be provided if her ICD begins to countershock inappropriately?
  - A medical magnet can be used to pause ICD function. (Remember that, when paused, the ICD will no longer manage any arrhythmias, so practitioners must be ready to manage these should they occur.)

- What are your goals for this patient?
  - Treat patient with supportive care.
  - Apply cardiac monitor for constant ECG monitoring.
  - Place defibrillation pads on patient's chest.
  - Deliver appropriate therapy.

- What are potential causes of inappropriate ICD firing?
  - Infection or erosion of the device. In most cases, the entire system must be removed.
  - Lead failure.
    - The leads are the weakest part of the ICD system, and the mechanical stresses on the leads can lead to breakage of the wires within the leads or in the insulation surrounding the leads.
  - Inappropriate detection and subsequent delivery of a shock.
  - Premature battery depletion or device failure.
    - Like any other piece of electronic equipment, these devices can occasionally fail without warning.
  - Improper sensing of an atrial arrhythmia with widened QRS.

She is transported in semi-Fowler position to the local hospital with a cardiac care center. She becomes more worried and anxious when placed in the ambulance. Therapeutic communication should be employed to keep the patient calm, as she is anxious her ICD will begin firing again. It is important to tell the patient that you cannot turn off the device. The patient is administered IV therapy and fluid at KVO, and continual ECG monitoring is performed. There are no changes on arrival at hospital.

CASE STUDY WRAP-UP

At the hospital, the cardiologist interrogates the ICD at her bedside, and it is determined that the ICD is not functioning properly (**FIGURE 15-9**). The patient consents to replacement of her malfunctioning ICD. A medical magnet is placed over the ICD and therapy electrodes are placed on her chest. She is brought to the cardiac intervention lab where a new ICD is placed. She was admitted to the cardiology ward where she is placed on telemetry to allow for constant ECG monitoring. She is discharged 3 days later with instructions to follow-up with her cardiologist.

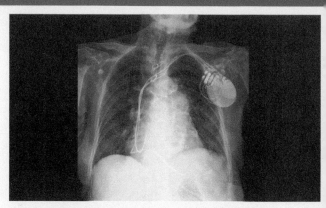

FIGURE 15-9 Radiograph of ICD in patient's chest.
© Yok_onepiece/Shutterstock

CHAPTER WRAP-UP

ICDs are used to identify and treat any potentially life-threatening arrythmia, including V-tach, V-fib, heart blocks, persistent severe bradycardias, and supraventricular tachycardias.

ICD patients can be recognized by medical ID bracelets or tags, a small rectangular shape beneath the skin on the left upper chest, and pacer spikes associated with widened QRS complexes on the ECG if the ICD is operating in pacemaker mode.

Treatment for a patient with an ICD is mainly comfort care following ICD discharge. These events are stressful for the patient and can generate reactions ranging from anxiety to post-traumatic shock injury after multiple shocks. The patient is required to consult with their cardiologist whenever the ICD discharges a countershock. Inappropriate shocks can be terminated by pausing ICD function. This is done through the placement of a donut-shaped medical magnet on top of the ICD.

REFERENCES

Lacour P, Parwani A. Are contemporary smartwatches and mobile phones safe with cardiovascular implantable electronic devices? *JACC Clin Electrophysiol.* 2020 Sep;6(9):1158–1166.

Sears S, Conti J. Quality of life and psychological functioning of ICD patients. *Heart.* 2002;87(5):488–493.

GEMS Glossary

activities of daily living (ADLs) Basic personal care activities that include feeding oneself, walking, continence, toileting, dressing, and personal hygiene.

adjustment disorders A group of disorders that involve an emotional or behavioral reaction to a stressful event that is considered excessive to an otherwise expected reaction. The reaction often significantly interferes with daily functioning and symptoms/response varies by age. Older adults tend to exhibit more depressive symptoms.

advance directive Written document that expresses a patient's wishes regarding their medical care and is intended to guide medical decision making when the patient is no longer able to communicate their wishes. The document varies from jurisdiction to jurisdiction. It may also be referred as a living will or healthcare directive.

adverse drug event (ADE) Occurs when a patient is harmed by a drug.

altered mental status (AMS) Any decrease in normal level of wakefulness, change in mentation, or behavior that is not normal for a particular person.

angioedema A vascular reaction that may have an allergic cause and may result in profound swelling of the tongue and lips.

aortic regurgitation Occurs when the valve does not completely close when the ventricle relaxes, allowing blood to re-enter the ventricle after contraction from both the aorta and the left atrium instead of solely the left atrium.

aortic stenosis Occurs when the valve becomes unable to completely open during ventricular contraction, inhibiting blood flow out of the chamber.

arteriosclerosis The thickening and stiffening of arterial walls.

asthma-COPD overlap syndrome (ACOS) Occurs when symptoms of both asthma and COPD are present in a patient. ACOS is not a separate disease and symptoms often present more frequently than with asthma or COPD alone; reduced lung function is often a result.

atherosclerosis A type of arteriosclerosis involving a narrowing of the blood vessels; a condition in which the inner layer of the artery wall thickens while fatty deposits build up within the artery.

barriers to care Obstacles that limit or prevent people from accessing and receiving adequate health care; multiple barriers are often present, increasing the risk of poor health outcomes and health disparities. Examples include lack of health insurance, limited or no access to transportation, limited health care resources in the patient's geographic location, language, and financial difficulty.

BEFAST Mnemonic used to identify stroke signs, assessing for balance, eyes, face, arm, speech, and time. This tool can detect more than 95% of patients with ischemic stroke.

bereavement The time or state of experiencing mourning and grieving after a loss or death. The time period often depends on the degree of attachment a person had to the deceased.

cardiac resynchronization therapy A procedure to implant a pacemaker or ICD to help the heart's ventricles contract in a more organized and efficient way to improve blood flow out of the heart.

caregiver fatigue Stress experienced by those who are caregivers, as their focus is on the caring of others rather than themselves.

caregiver stress Also known as "caregiver fatigue"; can lead to caregiver burnout.

chemoreceptors Chemical receptors that sense changes in the composition of blood and body fluids. The primary chemical changes registered by chemoreceptors are those involving levels of hydrogen (H+), carbon dioxide (CO_2) and oxygen (O_2). These changes can contribute to the stimulation of breathing elicited by buildup of carbon dioxide in the bloodstream or metabolic acidosis.

cholangitis An infection in the gallbladder or entire biliary system.

Cincinnati Prehospital Stroke Scale (CPSS) A common stroke assessment tool used by prehospital practitioners, which consists of testing for facial droop, arm drift, and abnormal speech.

Cullen sign A hemorrhagic discoloration of the umbilical area due to intraperitoneal hemorrhage from any cause; one of the more frequent causes is acute hemorrhagic pancreatitis.

delirium An abrupt change in mental status secondary to an acute medical condition; generally reversible once the underlying acute process is corrected. May be characterized by confusion, disorientation, restlessness, incoherence, fear, anxiety, excitement, or other non-baseline mental states.

dementia The general term for a decrease in cognitive capabilities that causes interference with activities of daily life.

destination therapy (DT) Placement of a permanent device in patients with heart failure who are not eligible for a heart transplant.

diverticula Small bulging pouches that form in the weaker areas of the intestinal lining, especially in the colon.

diverticulosis Development of small, bulging pouches (diverticula) in the colon's mucosa and submucosa through weak layers in the musculature of the colon.

do not attempt resuscitation (DNAR) See "do not resuscitate (DNR) order."

do not resuscitate (DNR) orders Documents that specify the medical care to be performed should the patient suffer cardiac arrest. These documents are also referred to as do not attempt resuscitations (DNARs). DNRs/DNARs serve the same purpose and are used in identical situations. DNAR has been adopted in some jurisdictions to reflect the low success rate of resuscitation for these patients. Some jurisdictions have two types of DNR documents.

DOPE mnemonic A mnemonic developed to guide the ventilator operator efficiently through a troubleshooting process: **D**islodgement of the endotracheal tube; **O**bstruction; **P**neumothorax; **E**quipment.

durable power of attorney (POA) A legal document similar to a medical power of attorney (MPOA), as it can also designate a person to make medical decisions for an incapacitated patient.

epidural hematoma Arterial bleeding that collects between the skull and dura mater.

epilepsy A persistent abnormality in the brain causing recurrent seizures.

euvolemic hyponatremia An electrolyte imbalance occurring when total body water increases, but the body's sodium content stays the same.

facility-related maltreatment This form of elder maltreatment includes both neglect (inadequate housekeeping practices [e.g., food left on trays], foul odors, not resolving problems when identified) and abuse. Indications of possible maltreatment can also include inconsistencies in staff reports, medical records, or between staff and family statements, or an unwillingness to release medical records.

femoral head fractures Rare, severe fractures of the upper end (femoral head) of the femur; often the result of a fall, but also commonly caused by violent, high-energy trauma, such as motor vehicle collisions.

femoral neck fractures Specific type of intracapsular hip fractures and the most common hip fractures; associated with low-energy falls, most often seen in older adults. The junctional location makes the femoral neck prone to fracture.

functional ability The extent to which a person is capable of being who they want to be and participating in activities that they value, such as mobility, ADLs, independence, contributing to society, etc. Functional ability is made up of the relevant aspects of a person's life, their own intrinsic capacity to function in meaningful ways, and how these two characteristics interact with each other.

geriatric Term used for those aged 65 years and older, though no official age is established as age-related changes vary by individual.

Grey Turner sign A discoloration of the left flank classically associated with acute hemorrhagic pancreatitis.

glucometry Measurement of the concentration of glucose in blood.

grieving The emotional process of reacting to the personal loss of a loved one through death, which may include feelings of great sadness, anger, guilt, and despair.

guardianship A directive by a court that declares someone incompetent and appoints another person to make decisions on their behalf; can include healthcare decisions.

healthcare directive See "advance directive."

heatstroke The most severe form of heat illness; develops when the body loses its ability to regulate temperature.

hematochezia Passage of red blood through the rectum.

hypertensive emergency A state of emergency differentiated from hypertension by the presence of signs or symptoms of organ damage due to the elevated blood pressure.

hypervolemia Abnormally increased volume of circulating fluid in the body.

hypovolemia Abnormally decreased volume of circulating fluid in the body.

iatrogenic A disease state, condition, or adverse effect caused by medical treatment; it usually results from a mistake made in diagnosis or treatment.

In-hospital DNR Advance directive included in a patient's medical file that is only valid while the patient is admitted to the hospital identified by the file.

inspiratory expiratory ratio Refers to the duration of the inspiration of breath as compared to the duration of expiration of breath; written as I:E. Normal breathing involves twic the duration of exhalation than inhalation and would be written as 1:2.

intrinsic capacity The physical and mental capacities a person has available to use in daily life, including the ability to think clearly, sensory input (seeing, hearing, tasting, feeling, smelling), memory recall, and mobility.

invasive ventilation Ventilation provided through an endotracheal or tracheostomy tube.

kyphosis An excessive or exaggerated outward rounding of the upper back most commonly found in older adults due to weakness in the spinal bones, causing compression; also called "hunch back" or "round back."

living will See "advance directive."

macroglossia Large tongue.

medical orders for life-sustaining treatment (MOLST) Medical orders that dictate medical care for a patient. This document must be signed by an authorized medical practitioner to be valid.

medical power of attorney (MPOA) A legal document that assigns a person to make medical decisions on a patient's behalf when the patient is unable to express their desires.

mitral regurgitation Incomplete heart valve closure causing blood to flow backward into the left atrium.

mitral stenosis Narrowing of the heart valve opening.

mourning The process by which someone adapts to a death, which is unique to each individual.

nephrotoxins Toxic agents or substances that inhibit, damage, or destroy the cells and/or tissues of the kidneys.

noninvasive mechanical ventilation Ventilation provided through a mask over the mouth and nose or nose alone; does not use an advanced airway.

orthostatic hypotension A form of low blood pressure that occurs when standing after sitting or lying down, which can cause dizziness, lightheadedness, and fainting; also called "postural hypotension."

osteoarthritis Cartilage destruction within the joint; often referred to as a "wear-and-tear" condition.

osteoporosis Condition of loss of bone mass and strength, whereby bones become weak and brittle, leading to increased fracture risk.

out-of-hospital DNR (OOH-DNR) Advance directive intended for reference by EMS practitioners. In many states, EMS can honor only a valid OOH-DNR document, while other types of advance directives are for use in healthcare facilities.

palliative care Care focused on preserving a patient's day-to-day living and independence by reducing the severity of their symptoms; this differs from standard care as no curative care is sought or provided (though curative care may be provided concurrently). Also known as "comfort care."

peak flow Ventilator speed at which the tidal volume is delivered; settings range from 35 to >100 L/min.

peak inspiratory pressure The peak pressure generated during ventilation, which should never exceed 40 cm H_2O to avoid lung injury due to over-inflation.

peripheral edema Displaced fluid from the capillaries in the lower body settles in the lowest body parts, typically the lower legs.

peripheral neuropathy Damage to the nerves located outside of the brain and spinal cord that causes pain, weakness, and numbness and pain, usually in the hands and feet. Other body functions may also be affected, including digestion, urination, and circulation. There are many causes, with diabetes being one of the most common.

phantom shocks Sensations of receiving ICD shocks; the cause of this phenomenon is unknown, but the same management is required when an ICD has activated, as phantom shocks can only be differentiated from a cardioversion event after the ICD data have been downloaded and the ECG rhythm interpreted.

pharmacodynamics What a drug does to the body based on where and what receptors, enzymes, or other proteins a drug binds to and modifies in the body; it is *not* affected by the aging process.

pharmacokinetics What the body does to a drug; the absorption, distribution, metabolism, and excretion of medications; it *is* affected by the aging process.

physician orders for life-sustaining treatment (POLST) See "medical orders for life-sustaining treatment (MOLST)."

polydipsia Excessive thirst.

polyphagia Excessive hunger.

polypharmacy Regularly using multiple medications concurrently.

polyuria Excessive urination.

preload The mechanical state of the heart at the end of diastole. It reflects venous return and the stress or stretch on the ventricular wall.

Prinzmetal angina Chest pain at rest with transient ischemic electrocardiographic changes in the ST segment, caused by spasm(s) of the coronary arteries; also known as, "vasospastic angina" or "variant angina."

proximal femoral fracture Fracture that occurs within the hip region; common in older persons with osteoporosis and high risk of falls; also results from trauma.

psychomotor ability Motor action directly proceeding from mental activity; relating to the relationship between conscious cognitive processing and the resulting physical movement.

pulmonary edema The condition of circulatory fluid displacing air within the alveoli.

pump failure A condition of decreased cardiac output due to decreased myocardial contractility, which leads to the inability to maintain metabolic needs.

purpura rash A non-blanching purplish discoloration of the skin that occurs when blood vessels burst and blood collects under the skin.

Rapid Arterial oCclusion Exam (RACE) A stroke assessment tool used in the prehospital setting to identify stroke severity and strokes likely involving a large artery occlusion. The five items assessed are (1) facial palsy; (2) neurolinguistic dysfunction (specifically, aphasia or agnosia); (3) leg motor function; (4) arm motor function; and (5) head/gaze deviation. Each item is scored on ability to fully perform a task, ability to partially perform a task, or inability to perform a task. The tool is scored out of 9 with a perfect score being 0. A score of 5 or higher indicates the likelihood of large vessel occlusion.

residual lung volume The amount of air left in the lungs after fully exhaling.

rheumatoid arthritis A type of chronic arthritis and autoimmune disease where the immune system attacks the tissue lining the joints on both sides of the body, causing pain, swelling, stiffness, and loss of function in the joints.

sarcopenia The age-related progressive loss of muscle mass, strength, and function.

scoliosis An abnormal lateral curvature of the spine.

Seniors Without Families Team (SWiFT) A triage tool designed to assess older adult residents in a shelter with no caregivers available. This tool rapidly separates residents based on their independence in performing ADLs. Once separated, each group can be assigned appropriate evacuation accommodations.

SPLATT assessment A mnemonic for post-fall assessment that can be used to help prevent future falls.

S: Symptoms the patient had prior to the fall could identify a medical disorder which led to the fall. **P**: Previous falls suffered by the patient could identify a pattern of cause. **L**: Location of fall could identify hazards that caused the fall. **A**: Activity immediately prior to fall could identify need for assist devices or other form of support. **T**: Time of day could identify need for better lighting. **T**: Trauma that caused or resulted from the fall that can be corrected (could be physical or psychological).

ST-elevation myocardial infarction (STEMI) Anginal symptoms at rest that result in myocardial necrosis as identified by elevated cardiac biomarkers with ST-segment elevation on the 12-lead electrocardiogram. These attacks carry a substantial risk of death and disability and call for a quick response by a system geared for reperfusion therapy.

stoma A surgical opening in the body deliberately kept open for drainage or other purposes, such as an opening in the abdominal wall for a colostomy.

subarachnoid hematoma Blood that has collected in the subarachnoid space from an arterial aneurysm rupture.

subdural hematoma The collection of blood between the covering of the brain (dura) and the surface of the brain (the subdural space).

tendinopathy Condition of tendon pain, swelling, and loss of function during an activity.

tetany A symptom caused by electrolyte imbalances where involuntary muscle contractions occur, as well as overly stimulated peripheral nerves. Low blood calcium levels (hypocalcemia) are most often to blame.

tidal volume A ventilator setting indicating the volume of air delivered with each ventilation; set at approximately 6 to 8 ml/kg of ideal patient weight.

toxidrome A constellation of signs and symptoms caused by exposure to a class of toxin.

unstable angina A progressive deterioration of angina (chest pain) in which the predictability of symptom onset is no longer reliable.

vital lung capacity The maximum volume of air that can be expired following maximum inspiration.

Index